ADHD: Attention-Deficit Hyperactivity Disorder in Children and Adults

ADHD: Attention-Deficit Hyperactivity Disorder in Children and Adults

■

Paul H. Wender, M.D.

OXFORD
UNIVERSITY PRESS
2000

OXFORD
UNIVERSITY PRESS

Oxford New York
Athens Auckland Bangkok Bogotá Buenos Aires
Calcutta Cape Town Chennai Dar es Salaam
Delhi Florence Hong Kong Istanbul Karachi
Kuala Lumpur Madrid Melbourne Mexico City
Mumbai Nairobi Paris São Paulo
Singapore Taipei Tokyo Toronto Warsaw

and associated companies in
Berlin Ibadan

Copyright © 2000 by Paul H. Wender

Published by Oxford University Press, Inc.
198 Madison Avenue, New York, New York 10016

Library of Congress Cataloging-in-Publication Data

Wender, Paul H., 1934–
    ADHD : attention-deficit hyperactivity disorder in children and adults /
Paul H. Wender.
    p. cm.
    Includes index.
    ISBN 0-19-511348-9 (alk. paper) — ISBN 0-19-511349-7 (pbk. : alk. paper)
    1. Attention-deficit hyperactivity disorder. 2. Attention-deficit-disordered
children. 3.Attention-deficit-disordered adults. 1. Title: Attention-deficit
hyperactivity disorder in children and adults. II. Title.

RJ506.H9 W448 2000
616.85'89—dc21

                                                        00-041671

3   5   7   9   8   6   4   2
Printed in the United States of America
on acid-free paper

Contents

■

Preface

■

To avoid possible confusion in terminology, let me explain what this book is about. Attention-Deficit Hyperactivity Disorder (ADHD) has had several names in the past. Among the earlier names were "minimal brain dysfunction," "hyperactivity," and Attention–Deficit Disorder (ADD). The latest and what we hope is the final name is Attention–Deficit Hyperactivity Disorder (ADHD). My earlier books about ADHD used its earlier names, "minimal brain dysfunction" and "hyperactivity."

In 1973, I published the first version of this book, *The Hyperactive Child*. During several years of treating "hyperactive" children, I had discovered that the parents of such children needed information about the nature, causes, and treatment of "hyperactivity," and that no book was available with such information in a form suitable for the concerned layperson. *The Hyperactive Child* was written in response to this need, drawing on clinical and research experience as previously summarized in a book for physicians and other professionals working with children (P. H. Wender, *Minimal Brain Dysfunction in Children*. New York: Wiley, 1971).

In 1978, the second version of the book was published that contained new information about the medical and psychological management of "hyperactivity." It also included a discussion of the learning disabilities that frequently—but not always—accompany hyperactivity.

In 1986, the third version was published. It was written for two reasons. One, as a continuing update. Two, to acquaint readers with "hyperactivity" in adults. It was based on information accumulated by my colleagues and myself on research on "hyperactivity" in adults that we had initiated in 1975. I felt that an understanding of the condition was as essential for ADHD adults as it was for the parents of ADHD children. The third edition presented what we had learned about the symptoms, the diagnosis, and the treatment of ADHD in adults.

This fourth edition, again, presents an update of our knowledge of ADHD in children, but it also presents a much greater expansion of what we have learned about ADHD in adults in our last fifteen years of research. It examines what we have discovered about the symptoms and the characteristic problems that ADHD adults experience socially, vocationally, and interpersonally and provides two rating scales we have developed for adults. These scales help determine if the adult had ADHD as a child and they also include the symptoms we use to determine whether he or she has continuing symptoms of ADHD. I have also included a screening rating scale that parents may fill out to determine whether their now adult children may have ADHD. The book also contains an update of our knowledge of drug and psychological treatments. Finally, I have included some case histories of ADHD children and ADHD adults so that the reader may get a more intimate feeling for the lives and experiences of the patients we treat.

This book is dedicated to the ADHD children and their families who have taught me so much about the disorder. It is dedicated also to those ADHD adults who have educated me about their problems and have willingly participated in scientific experiments over the past twenty-five years, experiments that have taught all of us more about ADHD in adults. I continue to believe that better understanding will lead to better treatment of ADHD and learning disabilities, frequently misunderstood disorders of childhood, adolescence, and adulthood.

P. W.

Salt Lake City, Utah
February 2000

ADHD: Attention-Deficit Hyperactivity Disorder in Children and Adults

1

Introduction

■

"Phil, stop acting like a worm,
The table's not a place to squirm"
Thus speaks the father to the son,
Severely says, not in fun.
Mother frowns and looks around,
But Philip will not take advice,
He'll have his way at any price.
He turns,
And churns,
He wiggles
And giggles
Here and there on the chair;
"Phil, these twists I cannot bear."
(After which he leans backwards in his chair, and as he is
   falling grabs
the tablecloth, tumbling him, the dishes, and the chair to
   the floor.)

"Fidgety Phil," translated from a German nursery rhyme,
   1863

Probably as many as four million children and four to five
million adults in the United States suffer from Attention-

Deficit Hyperactivity Disorder (ADHD). Although ADHD was described by physicians many years ago, its frequency only recently has been recognized. Exact figures are not available, but it seems likely that between 3 to 10 percent of school-age children and 4 to 5 percent of adults have ADHD. ADHD is frequently accompanied by learning disorders in reading, spelling, or arithmetic, and it may be accompanied by other behavior disorders. ADHD is more common in boys than in girls. Child psychiatrists used to believe that the symptoms of ADHD diminished and disappeared as children grew older, but recent studies have found that ADHD frequently persists into adolescence and adult life.

ADHD is the most recent term given by psychiatrists to a childhood disorder that has had a variety of names in the past. This disorder was first termed "hyperactivity," then "Attention-Deficit Disorder" (ADD), and then, to differentiate between children who had ADD but did not exhibit hyperactivity, either (plain) ADD or ADD-H. The new "official" term, Attention-Deficit Hyperactivity Disorder (ADHD), has been chosen by psychiatric experts, and its symptoms have been published by the American Psychiatric Association in its *Diagnostic and Statistical Manual of Mental Disorders* (DSM-IV). The definitions in this manual are widely acknowledged and are used among doctors, in research, and administratively for purposes of insurance. The earlier term, ADD, survives in the name of a major parent and patient support group, C.H.A.D.D.

Along with an increasing awareness of the problem of ADHD, a better understanding of its causes and treatment has developed. The purpose of this book is to explain to parents the present thinking about the nature of this problem and how to manage it. The book should, of course, be an aid—not a substitute—for diagnosis and treatment by a qualified physician. It is designed to answer many of the most frequently asked questions and to describe some of the simple procedures that many parents have found helpful in dealing with their ADHD children. It is also designed to help answer questions about the problems of ADHD and to describe treatments that have proven effective.

Although the behavioral problems that make up ADHD and the academic problems associated with learning disorders often occur together in the same person, it is useful to view each disorder separately. First, not all those with ADHD have the problems in reading, spelling, or arithmetic that are seen in learning-disordered people, and not all those with learning disorders have behavioral problems. Second, the treatment of ADHD behavioral problems and the treatment of learning disorder problems are different. For the most part, therefore, I will discuss them separately. Two behavioral disorders may accompany ADHD, Oppositional Defiant Disorder and Conduct Disorder, and I will discuss them briefly in Chapter 2.

The following are the most important points I want to make about ADHD.

1. ADHD is the most common chronic (ongoing) psychiatric disorder of childhood. It is probably two to three times more frequent in boys than in girls.

2. ADHD very frequently persists into adolescence and adulthood. Without treatment the ADHD child is likely to have increasing school difficulties and is much more likely than his non-ADHD classmate to develop behavioral problems that can lead to "at-risk" behavior—at risk to himself and to society, and, therefore, in the extreme, in the eyes of the law.

3. ADHD is not a recent discovery. "Fidgety Phil" has been around since 1863, and a British physician recognized ADHD symptoms in children at the beginning of this century. The use of medication to treat ADHD is also not new. A class of drugs called the amphetamines—Dexedrine® (d-amphetamine) or Desoxyn®

(methamphetamine)—was first used in the late 1930s. These drugs, still available, are every bit as effective overall as is the more commonly known drug, Ritalin® (methylphenidate).

4. ADHD is likely transmitted genetically, meaning it is probably a hereditary disorder. Exactly how it is passed on is not known, but it may be as a different structure or chemical functioning in the brain.

5. ADHD often occurs with other disorders. The most common ones are learning disorders and behavioral disorders, such as Oppositional Defiant Disorder and Conduct Disorder.

6. It is important to identify and treat ADHD as soon as possible for two reasons. First, treatment helps the child *now*. If the child learns more easily at school, it helps him avoid the anxiety and depression associated with academic difficulties, unpopularity with other children, and conflicts with his parents. Second, early treatment may decrease the risks of problem behavior ADHD children are more likely to develop in adolescence.

7. The diagnosis of ADHD in children is made on the basis of a careful history from the mother and father or others who have helped raise the child, an interview with the child, and from rating scales (used to describe the presence, frequency, and severity of symptoms) filled out by teachers and others who have worked with the child. The diagnosis of ADHD in adults is made on the basis of accounts by both the adult and someone close to the adult—a spouse or partner.

8. There are no special psychological or laboratory *tests* for determining whether a child has ADHD. As previously mentioned, the diagnosis is based on the interviews described and by rating scales. Although no special psychological or laboratory tests can diagnose ADHD, there *are* tests to diagnose learning disorders:

IQ tests and achievement tests in reading, spelling, and mathematics.

9. In many instances medication can reduce and sometimes eliminate many of the problems of ADHD in children, adolescents, and adults. Treatment with medication may produce substantial benefit in 70 percent of school-age children and in at least 60 percent of adults with ADHD. An important point about the drugs used to treat ADHD is that they are not addictive in ADHD patients when taken in the doses prescribed. A second point is that the treatment controls the symptoms of ADHD even though it does not *cure* it. This is not unusual in medicine. For example, insulin does not cure diabetes, but it enables diabetics to metabolize carbohydrates; anticonvulsants do not cure epilepsy, but they prevent epileptic seizures.

10. Psychological treatment of ADHD can be very helpful for both children and adults. Changes in child-rearing behavior can help parents deal with the ADHD child. Educational remediation (special education or resource education classes) may be useful for ADHD children who also have learning disorders. Currently these treatments are being evaluated in a large collaborative study conducted by the National Institutes of Mental Health.

11. In adulthood, medication is effective, and studies have shown that such therapies as couple therapy and psychoeducational therapy may be helpful. Others forms of treatment (such as group therapy) are being evaluated.

This book attempts to summarize what I have observed and learned in treating hundreds of ADHD children over a period of more than thirty-five years and what my colleagues and I have learned about ADHD from treating and doing research on several hundred adults during the past twenty-five years. In addition, it summarizes information obtained from the medical literature on the experiences and findings of other physicians. After describing the characteristics of children with ADHD, I will present current thinking on its causes. The changing nature of the disorder as the child matures will next be described, followed by a discussion of treatment, both medical and psychological. The persistence of ADHD into adulthood is then examined, along with its treatment. Finally, for both parents of ADHD children and for ADHD adults I will list sources of professional help in diagnosis and treatment.

In covering the subject of ADHD, I will use the following words many times: "few," "some," "frequently," "many," and "most." In medicine and education one can rarely use such words as "always," "every," or "never." The variety in people is stimulating in everyday life but complicating in medicine. Physicians would like to be able to use the words "always" or "never," but seldom can. This may make approaching the subject more difficult, but it will present a more realistic picture. To avoid awkward changes back and forth, I have used the pronoun "he" rather than "she." Similarly, I have used the word "spouse" rather than the more roundabout "significant other."

2

The Characteristics of Children with Attention-Deficit Hyperactivity Disorder

■

The task of describing the characteristics of children with Attention-Deficit Hyperactivity Disorder (ADHD) is in some ways a difficult one. The attributes are not unusual, but many of the symptoms are present in all children and adults to some degree at some particular time. Consequently, the parents reading this chapter are apt to conclude that all their children have ADHD. Before beginning, therefore, let me emphasize that the characteristics listed are not abnormal in themselves; they are only abnormal when they are excessive. What characterizes ADHD children is the *intensity*, the *persistence*, and the *patterning* of these symptoms. In this chapter I will also discuss other disorders that often occur in children with ADHD. This is important because they require different therapeutic approaches. Among the learning disorders are those associated with the areas of reading, spelling, or math. Studies have shown that somewhere between 20 to 30 percent of ADHD children have learning disorders. Among the psychological disorders are those classified as Oppositional Defiant Disorder (ODD) and Conduct Disorder (CD). Studies performed in clinics (where children are often referred by schools and social agencies) indicate that about 35 percent of ADHD children have ODD, and more than 25 percent have CD. Clinics are more likely to see severe cases of ADHD, however. Among ADHD children brought to private practitioners by parents, the rates of ODD and CD appear to be lower. (The DSM-IV criteria for ADHD, ODD, and CD can be found in Chapter 7, Finding Help.)

This chapter should not, of course, be used for diagnosis. It can, however, be used by a parent as a "screening" tool, as a help in deciding whether a child's behavior needs evaluating by a specialist. What the specialist can do is determine whether the child's symptoms are more severe than most children of that age and whether a problem exists. Only a clinician who has evaluated many children can accurately decide if a given child has ADHD. Parents who try to make the diagnosis alone are like medical students who, after reading the symptoms of diseases in their texts, think they have contracted smallpox, leprosy, and cancer within the space of a few weeks. (Fortunately, they recover just as rapidly.) Parents who suspect that their restless, poorly coordinated, distractible, and demanding child may have ADHD should seek the services of a competent specialist for diagnosis and a determination as to whether treatment is indicated.

Finally, I also want to emphasize that because the list of characteristics presented here is meant to be exhaustive, it will include some traits that are not necessarily present in all children with ADHD.

ATTENTION DIFFICULTIES AND DISTRACTIBILITY

One characteristic of the ADHD child that is almost always present is easy distractibility or shortness of attention span. This difficulty is not as obvious as hyperactivity but is of greater practical importance. The ADHD child does not have stick-to-itiveness. Young children, in comparison to adults, are relatively lacking in the ability to concentrate and follow through on long and tedious tasks. The ADHD child acts like a child younger than himself. He is the opposite of one who sits patiently in the corner painstakingly solving a puzzle and tolerating no interruptions. As a toddler and nursery school student, the ADHD child rushes quickly from activity to activity, and then seems at a loss for things to do. In school his teacher reports: "You can't get him to pay attention for long. . . . He doesn't finish his work. . . . He doesn't follow instructions." (And how could an inattentive child do so if the teacher says, "Take your geography book, turn to page 43, think about the first three questions, and write the answers in your workbook"?)

At home his mother notices that "he doesn't listen for long . . . he doesn't mind . . . he doesn't remember." The parents must hover over the child to get him to do what they want. Told once to eat with his fork and not his hands, he complies, but a few seconds later he is eating with his hands again. He may begin his homework as requested but fail to complete it unless the parents nag him. The child may not necessarily disobey instructions, but in the middle of an assigned job he starts doing something else. Tasks begun are half-done. His room is half-restored to order; the lawn is half-mowed. Sometimes, as discussed later, the child appears to remember but is reluctant to comply. Other times he appears to be distracted from the task at hand and forgets.

It is important to note that distractibility need not be present at all times. Often when the child receives individual attention he can attend well for a while. The teacher may report that he "does well with one-to-one attention." A psychologist may note that the child can pay attention during testing. A pediatrician may observe that the child was not inattentive during the brief office examination. They are all correct, but what is important is not how the child can pay attention when an adult is exerting the maximum effort to get him to do so. Many ADHD children can listen attentively for at least a little while. If the examiner, child psychiatrist, pediatrician, or psychologist does not realize the potential variability of such behavior, he or she may incorrectly come to the conclusion that the child is perfectly fine and that the parents and teacher are overreacting.

In *some* ADHD children, the distractibility may be concealed by the ability to stick with a particular activity for an unusually long period of time. Usually it is an activity they choose themselves. Sometimes it is a socially useful one (e.g., reading), and sometimes it is not. The child may seem to "lock on" and be undetachable or unusually persistent. The activity may be performed repetitiously for a long period of time. Such paradoxical behavior in an ostensibly distractible child may confuse a parent, who will ask, "How can he be distractible when he plays with his computer games for hours on end?" The highly unsatisfactory answer must be: "We do not know, but this is indeed the case."

HYPERACTIVITY

■

Not all ADHD children are hyperactive (which is the reason the name of the disorder was changed). However, most ADHD children are, and when hyperactivity is present it is very hard to miss. Many children with ADHD have been excessively active since early infancy. Parents often report that the child was "different" from the beginning of his life. Frequently, such infants are restless and have feeding problems and colic (intermittent and unexplained crying). They also often have sleeping problems of various sorts: some children fall asleep late and with difficulty, awaken frequently, and arise early; others fall asleep profoundly and are hard to arouse.

As these infants become toddlers, many of them are bundles of energy. Parents frequently report that after an active and restless infancy, the child stood and walked at an early age, and then, like an infant King Kong, burst the bars of his crib and marched forth to destroy the house. He was always on the go, always into everything, always touching (and hence, usually by mistake, breaking) every object in sight. When unwatched for a moment he somehow got to the top of the refrigerator or appeared in the middle of the street. In a twinkling, pots and pans were whisked from cupboards, glasses knocked off tables, and lamps overturned. The mother usually felt—and with good cause—that to take her eyes off him for one moment was to invite disaster: the moment her back was turned, something was broken or the toddler's life was in danger. And she was right. ADHD children have more than their share of accidents and are much more likely than non-ADHD children to be seen in emergency rooms.

As the ADHD child grows older the description changes: he is incessantly in motion, driven like a motor, constantly fidgeting, drumming his fingers, shuffling his feet. He does not stay at any activity long. He pulls all his toys off the shelf, plays with each for a moment, and then discards it. He cannot color for long. He cannot be read to without quickly losing interest. Of course he is unable to keep from squirming at the dinner table; he may not even be able to sit still in front of the TV. In the car he drives the other passengers wild. He opens and closes ashtrays, plays with the windows, tugs others' seat belts, and kicks the passengers in the front seat. At school his teacher relates that the child is fidgety, disruptive, unable to sit still; that he gets up and walks around the classroom, talks out, clowns; and that he jostles, bothers, and annoys his fellow pupils. Sometimes the ADHD child is as overtalkative as he is overactive, chattering as ceaselessly as he moves.

It is important to emphasize that what is different about the ADHD child is not his level of activity while at play. All children make all adults look like sloths. The ADHD child cannot be distinguished on the playground. His top speed is not greater than that of other children. What is so different about the ADHD child is that when he is requested to turn off his motor, he cannot do so for very long. Unlike other children, he cannot inhibit his activity in the home or the classroom. However, the ADHD child need not *always be* moving. Sometimes he can sit relatively still. For whatever reason, this is most apt to occur when he is getting individual attention from an adult. That is worth remembering because sometimes people who examine the child are misled when he sits more or less still for ten to fifteen minutes. They usually discover their error when they try to increase that time to an hour or so.

To repeat, an important point about ADHD is that *not all ADHD children are hyperactive*. There are ADHD children who have many of the problems I'm discussing but are not overactive at all, and there are even a few who are less than normally active. These ADHD children are more likely to be overlooked than those with hyperactive ADHD. This is particularly likely if they have learned to keep quiet as a way of avoiding embarrassment. *All the other problems can exist without hyperactivity itself.*

The second point is that clear-cut hyperactivity may be the first symptom to disappear as the child grows older. (However, it may simply remain in a less obvious form. The ADHD adolescent or adult may continually fidget or tap a foot and may describe himself as restless, unable to sit still for long, and prefer energetic to quiet activities.) Often the other problems persist. Therefore, even though the once overactive child has slowed down, not all problems are resolved. Many other problems may continue to require treatment even though the hyperactivity itself is gone.

IMPULSIVITY

■

A very frequently described characteristic of ADHD children is "impulsivity" or "poor impulse control." Every young child wants what he wants when he wants it. He acts without reflection or consideration of the consequences. The ability to tolerate delays, to count to ten, to think before acting, tends to develop with age. Again, the ADHD child behaves like a child several years younger than his chronological age.

He rapidly becomes upset when things or people fail to behave as he would have them behave. Toys get kicked (and sometimes broken), brothers and sisters and classmates are apt to get socked when they don't do what *they* should.

The ADHD child acts on the spur of the moment. He rushes into the street, onto the ledge, up the tree. As a result he receives more than his share of cuts, bruises, abrasions, and trips to the doctor. He wears out clothes or destroys toys— not maliciously but unthinkingly. It seemed like fun to walk in the street in his Sunday best; he wondered what would happen if he pulled that knob on the toy.

Impulsivity is also shown in poor planning and judgment. It is difficult to specify how much planning and judgment one should expect of children, but, again, ADHD children show less of these qualities than seems to be age appropriate. They are more likely than most children to run off in several directions at once. They are disorderly and disorganized. Their impulsivity combines with their distractibility to produce untidy rooms, sloppy dress (untucked shirts, unzipped zippers), unfinished assignments, careless reading and writing.

Another area that is a problem in some ADHD children is bladder and bowel control, and it may be related to their impulsivity. When younger, some ADHD children may wet or soil themselves slightly during the day. They seem to pay no attention to their "pressing needs" and overflow somewhat. Bed-wetting, which occurs in about 10 percent of all six-year-old boys, seems to be more common in ADHD children. It may be that bed-wetting in some ADHD children is related to unusually deep sleep, but this is not certain. The relationship between ADHD and bed-wetting is important to recog-

nize because "accidents" and bed-wetting are sometimes assumed to be a sign of anatomical abnormalities or deep
psychological problems. Often, however, they are instead a
manifestation of ADHD and respond to the general treatment
prescribed for it.

Social impulsivity—antisocial behavior—is *sometimes* a
problem in ADHD children. At some time all children steal,
all children lie, most children play with matches. As they
grow older most children learn to inhibit these impulses. A
few ADHD children do not; they take, lie, or light matches
whenever they want to. Now ADHD itself does not explain
why children wish to do these things. Children steal for a
wide variety of reasons. Stealing may result from a simple
desire to have or from a desire to have things that would buy
affection; it may be an attempt to achieve status in a group;
it may be a source of excitement; or it may be a means of
retaliating or obtaining attention or punishment. What is important is that if these motives occur in the ADHD child, he
is less able than other children to control himself. It should
be obvious that treatment of such a child would require a
twofold approach: dealing with the specific motivation and
reducing the impulsivity (or increasing the ability for self-
control).

And, as with hyperactivity, impulsivity may not be present. The ADHD child may only be inattentive. This is important because, like hyperactivity, impulsivity is very noticeable while inattention may not be. The ADHD child may
"only" have problems with inattention and distractibility,
but we often find that these symptoms "alone" can cause
difficulties not only at school but also in his relations with
other children. The inattentive child may miss the point of
a story another child is telling and interrupt. He is then
thought of as "out of it" by his peers. Or the child may miss
instructions for a game and make mistakes. One soccer coach
I know insists that his ADHD player take his medicine before the start of a game.

ATTENTION-DEMANDING BEHAVIOR

In order to develop normally, all children require adult interest, involvement, and attention. As they grow older, they require less but still need the awareness and interest of those whom they love and respect.

The ADHD child demands attention, but this in itself is not what makes him different. He is different and difficult because of his insatiability. Like a younger child he wants to be always on center stage. He may whine, badger, tease, and annoy without stopping. The manifestations change with age. As a toddler he may repeat annoying and prohibited activities; as an older child he may attempt to monopolize the dinner-table conversation, clown in the classroom, and show off with his friends at some risk and to the distress of law enforcement agencies.

These aspects of his behavior may be concealed by the fact that he sometimes does not manifest certain kinds of affectionate behavior. Many, although far from all, ADHD children have been undemonstrative. In infancy they were noncuddlers. They did not go to sleep on laps but wiggled off to go about their own business. They were not upset when their mothers left them with babysitters or at nursery school. Nonetheless, the same children sometimes figuratively managed to stand at arm's length and prod their parents with a pole.

The demand for attention can be distressing, confusing, and irritating to parents. Since the child demands so much, they feel they have not given him what he needs. Because they cannot understand how to satisfy him, they feel deficient. Finally, because the child may cling and poke simultaneously and endlessly, they feel angry.

SCHOOL DIFFICULTIES AND
LEARNING DISORDERS

■

In discussing the school difficulties that sometimes afflict ADHD children, it is important to emphasize that ADHD does *not* affect intelligence as ordinarily defined and measured by intelligence tests. The proportions of the bright, normal, and slow are the same among ADHD children as among children who do not have ADHD. Attention-Deficit Hyperactivity Disorder is not in any way related to mental retardation.

However, *some* ADHD children, not all, do have certain problems in intellectual development. Some may have an "unevenness" of intellectual development. Intelligence tests measure abilities and skills in a number of separate areas, such as vocabulary, arithmetic, understanding, memory, and certain forms of problem solving. Usually a child's performance is pretty much the same in each of these separate areas. If a child's vocabulary is normal for his age, his memory and problem solving are usually age-normal as well. ADHD children may be more likely to have uneven development. Thus, an ADHD child's intelligence, which averages his ability in all these areas, may be average yet he may be advanced in some and behind in others. This can produce difficulties in school placement and adjustment. An ADHD child in the third grade may be able to do fifth-grade mathematics but only second-grade reading. If the school does not make allowances for these inconsistent abilities, the problems of such a child will be accentuated. He cannot be moved to a regular fifth or second grade, for he will be too slow for one and too fast for the other. Unless the school can arrange a program to take his abilities into account, he will not fit into *any* class.

As I indicated earlier, ADHD is frequently accompanied by

Learning Disorders (LD), a term used to describe difficulty in reading, spelling, or math. The formal diagnostic names are reading disorder, spelling disorder, and mathematics disorder. All children (and adults) with LDs have problems performing in one or more of these academic areas despite normal intelligence, adequate teaching, and absence of psychiatric illness. Learning Disorders are classified as developmental disorders because children with them fail to acquire these skills as they grow and mature. We do not use the term reading disorder for children who are intellectually slow in many areas, including reading. Such children are equally and predictably slow in a wider range of areas, so that one would expect them to have difficulty in reading. Individuals with LD have a discrepancy between their intelligence and their performance in reading and/or spelling and/or arithmetic. For example, consider a ten-year-old third grader with average intelligence. He should be reading at a ten-year-old level. If the child is only reading as well as an average eight year old, he is two years behind and may be diagnosed as having a developmental disorder in reading.

Two questions about LD are usually asked by parents. The first is "How can a child get a normal score on an intelligence test and have trouble with reading?" The answer is that the kind of intelligence tests that are used to diagnose suspected LD do not involve reading. The psychologist *asks* questions of the child, and the test is designed to measure such things as knowledge, abstraction, reasoning, memory, problem solving, observational ability, and quickness. We do not know enough about the brain and mind to know why someone can be very smart and yet be unable to read well or to add up a column of numbers, but we do know that many such people exist. I have seen children and adults with marked LD who read painfully slowly or who cannot add figures in their checkbook (or in scientific experiments!) but who play a brilliant game of chess, are sophisticated inventors, or are at home in advanced mathematics. Such uneven development has important practical consequences, of course, both for education and for the psychological well-being of the person with an LD.

The second question usually asked is "How far behind does someone have to be to be diagnosed as having a LD?" There is no scientific reason for selecting a particular number, but generally school systems say two years. Thus, LDs are often not definitely diagnosed until the third grade. Then, if a child is two years behind, he can be identified as reading like a normal first grader. However, although it is difficult to diagnose LDs before the third grade, parents and teachers are often correct in suspecting such problems when the first- or second-grade child is lagging far behind the other children in learning to read.

In developmental reading disorder one sees difficulties in reading out loud, together with adding, omitting, and changing words. In spelling to dictation there are frequent errors. Letters may be reversed ("b" confused with "d") or transposed. Handwriting is often horrendous—illegible and unplanned, wandering all over the page. Children with an LD in arithmetic often reverse figures in columns and show difficulties with word problems (if apples cost three cents each and I buy eight and give you a quarter, how much do you owe me?). In addition to these relatively specific problems, children with LDs may have various other problems, such as difficulty in telling right from left. One patient with right/left difficulties solved his problem by putting his watch on his left hand—and he remembered the left hand because it was the one with the mole! Some have trouble with spatial relations—the person cannot follow directions to find his way around a strange place or city. Sometimes the child has difficulty in learning sequences (such as the days of the week or the months of the year) or in telling time (before the invention of the digital watch). For others, learning and retaining the multiplication table present special problems.

Some experts who have studied LD think that problems in reading can usefully be thought of as falling into different categories. One well-known investigator, Elena Boder, has suggested a tentative two-part classification that many workers in the field find helpful. Boder divides LD children into two overlapping groups: auditory-language dyslexics (A-dyslexics) and visual-spatial dyslexics (V-dyslexics). The A-dyslexic has a good visual memory but has difficulty with phonetics—that is, he has trouble relating isolated sounds and the small groups of letters on the printed page that refer to syllables. If he knows a word, he knows it as a whole. He will be able to read and spell words that he has previously mastered. But because he has not grasped phonetics he has trouble in reading and spelling unfamiliar words.

The V-dyslexic understands phonetics. He can sound out new words and, if they are phonetic, he can often do so correctly. Similarly, he will spell unfamiliar words phonetically. However, he has a higher than normal number of letter and word reversals and omissions.

Boder believes that A-dyslexia is four to five times as common as V-dyslexia, although many children have a mixture of both problems. She believes that other problems are specifically associated with A- and V-dyslexia. For example, she finds that A-dyslexics tend to do better in problem solving than in verbal parts of intelligence tests, and that V-dyslexia is sometimes accompanied by difficulty in distinguishing between right and left and by poor handwriting.

I cannot emphasize too much that it is possible to have these problems and still be intelligent. Many fine athletes, musicians, and mechanics have LDs. There are numerous ways in which children and adults with LDs can compensate for their deficiencies. Eminent people known for high achievement have had LDs—for example, Thomas Edison and Harvey Cushing (the father of neurosurgery) had severe dyslexia. Academic skills represent only one part of the vast range of human skills and they have become more important only recently, as literacy has become widespread.

It is useful to compare people with LDs with tone-deaf

people. Tone-deaf people generally have normal hearing and normal intelligence but have difficulty in reproducing musical pitch accurately. They have trouble, for example, singing in tune or playing the violin. Everyone understands that one can be very intelligent and yet be unable to carry a tune. If singing were important and reading were not—as in some primitive tribes—tone-deaf people would be handicapped as if they had an LD. In hunting societies, speed and coordination would be the most important skills; dyslexia (and tone deafness) would be irrelevant. Thus dyslexia is a culture-dependent disorder.

Nevertheless, we must not underestimate the importance of these LDs, which we think are physically produced. Having trouble in reading or arithmetic not only makes progress difficult in the academic and business worlds but also leads to typical psychological problems. I will return to these problems in later chapters.

Remember that many ADHD children do not have LDs. Nevertheless, most ADHD children have considerable difficulty in learning at school. "Underachievement" is almost a hallmark of the ADHD child and adolescent. Teachers and guidance counselors will, of course, recognize that the child has problems, and sometimes the school is the first place that the child's problems are clearly recognized. However, school personnel sometimes underestimate the problems related to ADHD and may attribute the child's difficulties to emotional problems, psychological maladjustment, or problems in the home.

If the ADHD child does *not* have specific LDs, there are several possible explanations for his poor school performance. All his learning problems may stem from the attention difficulties and emotional overreactivity that are also discussed in this chapter. An eight year old with ADHD, despite normal intelligence, may be reacting to the school in the same fashion as a normal four or five year old. Intelligence is not enough. A child must have the ability to concentrate for a reasonable period of time; he must hear at least *some* of what is said if he is to learn. He must have a reasonable amount of stick-to-itiveness and patience to tolerate difficult tasks; if he gives up immediately, learning will obviously be impaired. And, as has been mentioned several times, the ADHD child is both inattentive and readily frustrated. The learning problems are further complicated because they tend to move in vicious circles; they often snowball. His poor performance is apt to cause the teacher to say, either in so many words or indirectly: "Why can't you use your brains? . . . Why don't you finish your work? . . . Do your work. . . . You could if you wanted to." Thus, poor performance leads to criticism, which in turn leads to the child's having a poor opinion of himself. Both are likely to decrease his motivation to do well. If he can't do well when he is trying to the best of his ability, he tends to give up. The result is a performance that grows steadily worse. If a child is a bit slow in the first few grades, he remains at a disadvantage even if most of the ADHD disappears and his learning ability catches up. Since he is now behind academically, school is harder and most frustrating.

Finally, much of any school experience is boring, tedious, and repetitious. Many parents who visit an elementary school for the first time in ten or twenty years are impressed with its tedium and wonder how they were able to pay attention when they were children. This is not to say that making school into a consistently interesting experience would eliminate the ADHD child's difficulties. Probably it would not. I only mean to point out that the social structure in most schools makes the ADHD child's problems greater.

DIFFICULTIES IN COORDINATION

■

Approximately half of ADHD children show various difficulties in coordination. Some ADHD children have limited "fine-motor control": they have trouble coloring, cutting with scissors, tying shoelaces, and buttoning. Handwriting is often terrible and the ADHD child perceives writing as a chore. The combination of poor coordination and failure to plan can lead to an illegible written page, with words overrunning lines, the sides of the page, and each other. Others may have some mild difficulty with balance—for example, in learning to ride a bicycle. Still other ADHD children may have poor hand-eye coordination: these children will be awkward in throwing and catching a ball or in playing baseball or tennis. Not all ADHD children have such problems. Many are well coordinated and some are excellent athletes. When coordination problems are present, they usually cause more difficulties for boys than for girls because for boys athletic ability is an important source of acceptance by others. However, even the children with coordination handicaps may have no problems in activities requiring large muscle groups and may run or swim without difficulty.

RESISTANT, OPPOSITIONAL, AND DOMINEERING SOCIAL BEHAVIOR

■

Most hyperactive children manifest interpersonal behavior that has several distinct characteristics: (1) a considerable resistance to social demands, a resistance to "do's" and "don'ts," to "shoulds" and "shouldn'ts"; (2) increased independence; (3) domineering behavior with other children.

Probably the single most disturbing feature of ADHD children's behavior, and the one most frequently responsible for their referral for treatment, is the difficulty many of these children have in complying with requests and prohibitions of parents and teachers. Some ADHD children may appear almost impossible to discipline. In some respects they seem to remain two years old. Parents describe them as "obstinate . . . stubborn . . . negativistic . . . bossy . . . disobedient . . . sassy . . . not caring." All the techniques of discipline seem unsuccessful: rewards, removal of privileges, physical punishment. "He wants his own way. . . . He never seems to hear. . . . He never learns by his own mistakes. . . . You can't reach him. . . . Punishment just rolls off his back. . . . He's almost immune to anything we do." ADHD children differ, however, in the ways they manifest resistance. Some seem to forget what they are told, whereas others seem to actively oppose what is requested of them. I will discuss the meaning of this when I discuss the causes of the disorder.

With regard to independence, the ADHD child is often excessively independent but in a few instances can be excessively dependent. The independence may be noticed at an early age. The ADHD child is the sort apt to wander ten blocks away from home when he is two years old. When he is brought home to his terrified and angry parents, he is smiling and excited. He does not seem to get upset by the separation. He is *not* the sort of child who is likely to be upset the first few days of nursery school or kindergarten or when left with his grandparents. The few ADHD children at the other extreme, those who are excessively dependent, tend to be immature, babyish, and clinging. They are the children most likely to show the incessant attention-demanding behavior that I have described.

The ADHD child's relationships with his brothers, sisters, and schoolmates are likely to follow a clearly recognizable pattern. When he is younger he tends to be a tease. He becomes quite expert at getting others' goats, annoying, and bothering. As he grows older, he shows a very marked tendency to be bossy. Note how this contrasts with his refusal to be bossed by adults. When he plays with other children he strives to be the leader. He wants to decide what games will be played. He wants to decide what the rules are and, if the game is not played the way he likes, he may quit: he wants to play it his way or not at all. Needless to say, this does not win friends and influence people (at least favorably). Other children tend to avoid him, and after a while the ADHD child is likely to be without friends. This lack of friendship is much different from what one sees in a shy, withdrawn child. The ADHD child is usually aggressive socially and *initiates* friendship successfully, but his style drives other children away. He will tell his parents that he is talked about, rejected, and perhaps even bullied. These reports are not excuses and they are not inaccurate. They are correct assessments of what his own behavior compels other children to do. He "makes friends easily but can't keep them." As a result, the ADHD child often plays with younger children. However, the ADHD child is not necessarily physically aggressive. He is not sadistic and does not enjoy hurting others. He *does* tend to have more than his share of fights, but this is because of his impulsivity and because brothers and sisters and schoolmates are usually not enthusiastic about being pushed around and told what to do.

EMOTIONAL DIFFICULTIES

■

Most ADHD children show certain forms of emotional problems. The word *emotional* is one of those vague terms used by everyone in a variety of ways whose meaning is not clear. Let me emphasize first that calling these problems emotional does *not* imply that they are psychologically caused—indeed, most of them are probably not.

ADHD children tend to have mood swings and cycles, so their behavior tends to be unpredictable. Parents report: "He's happy one minute, impossible to get along with the next. . . . He has his good days and bad days, and it's hard to understand why." The last statement is important. All of us have our good and bad days, and often we can link our moods to our experiences. In the case of the ADHD child, it is usually more difficult to find out why he was bad yesterday and good today.

Many ADHD children are unusually underreactive and overreactive. They are sometimes insensitive to pain. They seem unaffected by and rarely react to the frequent bumps, falls, and scrapes that are the lot of younger children. (This is sometimes obscured by increased attention-seeking. When their parents are looking they may tend to squeeze out every last drop of sympathy obtainable.) They are often relatively fearless. A combination of this fearlessness, a craving for attention, impulsivity, and a tendency not to "plan ahead" is apt to land them in socially unapproved situations: when young, at the tops of trees; when older, impressing their adolescent peers with taboo behavior and inviting the interest of the local police. Fortunately, such fearlessness is *not* seen in all ADHD children.

The overreactivity of ADHD children sometimes manifests itself in excessive excitement during pleasant activities. Most young children will be excited at the circus, but ADHD children tend to become quite overexcited in such circumstances. They may even lose control of themselves in less stimulating situations, for example, during a visit to a supermarket. This overreactivity can also be seen in excessive irritability or anger during frustrating activities. Of course, most children (and adults) do not tolerate frustration or disappointment very well. But the ADHD child has a much lower tolerance for frustration and a more violent reaction to it. When things do not go his way, he is subject to temper tantrums, angry outbursts, or sullen spells. Most young children become irritable and babyish when tired or hungry. An eight-year-old ADHD child may react to fatigue or hunger in the same way that a normal four year old does.

Although many parents describe their ADHD children as "angry," what they usually seem to be referring to is irritability and hot temper rather than aggressiveness or hostility—that is, hyperreactivity to comparative minor situations: "He's got a low boiling point . . . a short fuse. When he's angry he loses control." Many ADHD children are described as being good-natured except during such outbursts.

One other characteristic seen in some ADHD children that is frequently disturbing to parents might be called "unsatisfiability." "He never gets a kick out of anything, at least not for long. . . . He can't be bothered to do much, nothing really seems to give him pleasure . . . you can never satisfy him." This characteristic is sometimes produced by spoiling (in adults as well as children), but many ADHD children behave this way without ever having been spoiled. Their mothers may have noticed that they were not satisfiable from early infancy.

Finally, one "emotional" characteristic of most ADHD children is also found in many children with other difficulties: low self-esteem. They have little self-confidence: "He doesn't think much of himself. . . . He thinks he's bad. . . . He thinks he's different." The cause and the treatment of such low self-esteem are discussed at greater length later.

IMMATURITY

■

Immaturity is neither a very scientific nor a very specific word, but it often does accurately describe the behavior of ADHD children. Their lack of social, athletic, and academic skills, their inability to remember—and act on—"do's and don'ts" are certainly characteristic of younger children. The inability to tolerate frustration (often resulting in tantrums) and the lack of stick-to-itiveness are normal in younger children. Finally, *some* ADHD children have another trait associated with immaturity: rigidity, the inability to tolerate change (such children, for example, will be upset if their routine is changed or if the furniture in their room is rearranged). From a practical standpoint, it is often helpful for parents to remember that emotionally, *not* intellectually, their ADHD child may behave very much like a child four or five years younger. Remembering this often makes it easier for parents to handle their child; many parents do not know how to act toward a nine year old with problems but do know how to deal with a normal four or five year old. If the parents can remember that their ADHD nine year old is in *some* respects acting like a normal five year old, they may find it easier to understand and help him.

CHANGING PROBLEMS WITH AGE

A salient aspect of the ADHD child's problems is that they tend to change as he grows older. The behavioral problems that are conspicuous in a toddler are very different from those in an adolescent. There are several reasons for this. First, there seem to be changes associated with maturation; for example, the symptoms themselves tend to diminish with age (just as bed-wetting disappears with age). Second, some changes occur as a result of learning: the ADHD child is more hostile after his tenth year of rejection by schoolmates than he is after only one or two years of such treatment. Third, recognition of "problems" depends on one's understanding of the behavior considered normal for particular age groups: fidgety behavior is expected and tolerated in nursery school children but not in second graders; reading difficulty is expected in all first graders but is a problem in fourth grade.

What is the usual sequence of difficulties? In infancy the ADHD child's most conspicuous problems are in physiologic function: he is likely to be irritable, to have colic, and to have sleep disturbances. During the toddler stage his ability to do things increases immensely, and many of them are troublesome things. The most disturbing traits are his continual "getting into" things and his inability to listen—that is, to respond to parental discipline.

As he reaches preschool age, his problems with attention and social adjustment claim the limelight. His short attention span, low frustration tolerance, and temper tantrums make sustained play and nursery school participation difficult. Problems with his schoolmates soon appear: teasing, domination, and other annoying behaviors. These qualities endear him neither to his teacher nor to his fellows, and in a few instances result in his beginning his academic career as a kindergarten dropout.

When he starts the first grade, his restlessness attracts attention: his teacher complains that he cannot sit still, that he gets up and walks around, whistles, and shuffles. Academic problems, though often present, tend to be ignored. First graders are not expected to read immediately. Bed-wetting may now appear. Although he may have always been a bedwetter, bed-wetting is defined as a problem only when the child reaches an age when it is expected to disappear (usually about six), or when he stays overnight at camp or with friends. At about the third grade, when the child is nine or ten, academic and antisocial problems attract the most attention. Until that time slowness in school can be attributed to immaturity or academic unreadiness. But in the third grade the diagnosis is changed to learning problems or learning disability. Reading difficulty causes the greatest concern, but the child may also have trouble with arithmetic and be criticized for messy writing. Outside of school, antisocial behavior is likely to be the cause of considerable concern. Both the duration and intensity of these problems are highly variable.

If the problems persist into early adolescence, the antisocial problems become the focus of attention. If academic problems persist, they may now be taken for granted. This is not to say that the same child who has a reading problem predictably develops social problems. Rather, if the child has both reading and social problems, the social problems attract the greatest concern at this time.

I wish to emphasize very strongly that the age patterns I have described do not apply to all ADHD children. Some children manifest difficulties in all developmental stages, some in only a few. At any one stage, the difficulties vary from child to child: some will have academic problems, some will have coordination problems, some will have learning problems, some will have social problems, some will have different combinations of these problems, and an unfortunate few will have all of them.

Finally, many ADHD children tend to outgrow not only their hyperactivity but also a large proportion of the associated other difficulties. Any given ADHD child may follow the developmental sequence listed and then may no longer manifest ADHD characteristics at a later stage, say, as a preadolescent.

The combination of problems that are seen among ADHD children constitutes what is called a *syndrome* in medical terminology. A syndrome is a group of difficulties that *tend* to clump, cluster, or move together. It is characteristic of medical syndromes for a given individual not to have all the problems associated with the syndrome. For example, some ADHD children may have problems primarily with inattention and distractibility without the other symptoms I have discussed (See Appendix), while most will have problems with inattention and distractibility together with many of the symptoms I have mentioned. These children are frequently overlooked because their behavior in school, daydreaming or woolgathering, is not disruptive and is less likely to attract teachers' attention and therefore remain undiagnosed. This is unfortunate because these children are likely to be underachievers in school and because it appears that they are responsive to the same treatment that is so helpful for ADHD children with the additional symptoms that are described in the rest of this chapter. It is also important to note that the child who does not have some of the problems listed at any given stage in his development is very unlikely to develop them at a later stage. The child who does not have coordination problems when he is young will not get them when he is older. The child who does not have reading problems when he is seven or eight will not have them as a teenager. To the parents burdened with those difficulties that their ADHD child does have, this optimistic aspect of his development may be of some comfort. It is not to be minimized, for it has been observed by physicians who have treated these children and worked with their families over periods of years.

Unfortunately, the syndrome of ADHD does not prevent the occurrence of other psychiatric disorders. The ADHD child who turns resistant behavior into defiant behavior may be classified as having the accompanying disorder, Oppositional Defiant Disorder (ODD). This disorder is described as a "recurrent pattern of negativistic, defiant, disobedient, and hostile behavior toward authority figures." He will often lose his temper, argue with adults, actively defy their requests, deliberately do things to annoy others, and be angry and resentful or spiteful and vindictive. When these symptoms exist alongside ADHD, the child is described as ADHD-ODD. A more pronounced disorder is Conduct Disorder (CD), and it too may be seen in some ADHD children (who would then be described as ADHD-CD). The relationship is important: only *some* ADHD children have CD, but most children with

CD have ADHD. CD children's core problem is "a repetitive and persistent pattern of behavior in which the basic rights of others or major societal norms or rules are violated. Such children are aggressive, destructive of property, and lie and steal." About half of CD children continue to behave in a similar way as adults. ADHD with CD is more severe than ADHD alone, and most clinicians believe it should be treated vigorously at an early age. Other disorders may be present, such a major mood disorders or anxiety disorders, but it is not clear whether there is an increased frequency among ADHD children. The important point is to bring to the attention of a clinician the behavior that is causing the child difficulties with those around him.

For those ADHD children who do continue to have problems related to the disorder in adolescence and adulthood, research suggests that a combination of the various treatments available for ADHD may lead to a better prognosis. I will describe in greater detail what is known about ADHD in adolescents and adults in later chapters.

3

The Causes of Attention-Deficit Hyperactivity Disorder

■

The majority of cases of attention-deficit hyperactivity disorder appear to be *genetically transmitted* and *chemically produced*. Stating it differently, attention-deficit hyperactivity disorder seems to be hereditary and what is inherited is abnormal chemical functioning within the brain. Stimulant drugs, the most effective treatment for ADHD, most probably have a normalizing effect, correcting the imbalances that are believed to produce ADHD.

How the child is treated and raised can affect the severity of his problem, but it cannot cause the problem. Certain types of raising may make the problem worse; certain types may make the problem better. No forms of raising can produce ADHD problems in a child who is not temperamentally predisposed to them. Because child-rearing techniques can to some degree affect the seriousness of the ADHD child's problem, changes in these techniques are usually helpful. They will be discussed in Chapter 5 on treatment. Even though such psychological approaches can be helpful in the management of the ADHD child, this does not affect the explanation of the origin of the syndrome—the basic source of the difficulties seems to be inborn.

CAUSES OF THE
TEMPERAMENTAL PROBLEMS

∎

Recent scientific evidence supports what everyone's grand-mother knew: there are inborn temperamental differences among children. Studies of the growth of children from infancy to preadolescence reveal that children differ from their earliest days and that some of these differences tend to be associated with behavioral problems as the child grows up. For example, the difficulties that the ADHD child is likely to have in infancy (colic, feeding problems, sleeping problems) are probably the result of inborn temperamental differences. What causes these differences? Child psychiatrists are not certain. A very good possibility is that they are the result of chemical differences in the brain. The brain is an extraordinarily complex interconnection of nerve cells. In some ways it is analogous to a telephone network, but with one major difference. In the telephone network the connections are *electrical*; electricity passes from one wire to another by physical contact. In the brain, however, the connections are *chemical*. One nerve cell releases a small amount of certain chemicals, which are picked up by a second cell, causing it to "fire." These chemicals are called *neurotransmitters*. If there is too little of a particular neurotransmitter, the second cell will not fire because not enough of the neurotransmitter has been released by the first cell. Although the nerve cells themselves are intact, it's as if the connection were broken. There are different neurotransmitters in different portions of the brain. If the amount of one neurotransmitter is insufficient, the portion of the brain that it operates will not function correctly. ADHD children are probably deficient in some neurotransmitters. (In some ADHD children the quantity of these transmitters might increase with age.)

These presumed chemical differences are generally thought

to be inherited, part of the individual's genetic makeup. Could they also be the result of a misstep in the development of the baby before birth? That is, could ADHD be produced because the normal pattern of "wiring" in the brain or the chemistry of the brain has been altered? Little is known about prenatal influences, but there is some possibility that extremely small birth size—and therefore prematurity—may sometimes lead to ADHD symptoms. Similarly, other variations in the mother's biological processes during pregnancy might result in fetal maldevelopment. However, much more frequently, genetic origins have been observed. ADHD and reading problems have been noted to run in families. Other traits such as hair color, eye color, or certain forms of mental deficiency also tend to run in families, and these traits are related to the production of particular chemicals in the body. The amounts and types of these chemicals are determined by our genes. Certain genes may also control the amounts of neurotransmitters and some genes may result in decreased availability of these neurotransmitters. Neurochemists have some possible leads about which neurotransmitters may be insufficient in ADHD children. These chemicals are located in portions of the brain that includes among its functions the regulation of attention. An excess of these neurotransmitters might produce an increased ability to focus attention and inhibit behavior, to control oneself. A deficiency in these neurotransmitters—which is probably the condition present in ADHD children—would produce an underactivity of that portion of the brain, resulting in attention difficulties and some lack of self-control. These portions of the brain probably also act to modulate the mood and increase appropriate reactions to things going on outside the child. Therefore, decreased availability of neurotransmitters in this area would result in a decreased ability to focus attention; a decreased ability to check one's behavior—to apply brakes; a decreased sensitivity to others' reactions—to do's and don'ts, and approval or disapproval; and a decreased ability to modulate mood—that is, an increased tendency toward sudden and dramatic mood changes.

That ADHD is genetic is not surprising. It is a common observation that particular kinds of temperament tend to run in families. In some families the children are high-strung (like fox terriers or cocker spaniels), whereas in others the children are more placid (like basset hounds). Any temperamental characteristic is not an all-or-none trait. It is like height. There are all degrees of tallness, from the very short to the very tall. Most people who are very short or very tall do not suffer from a disease, although it may be very inconvenient to be 4' 6" or 7' 2". Similarly, most degrees of high-strungness do not cause problems unless they are excessive. All the traits of ADHD children that I have discussed occur in all children. At times, all children have short attention spans, are restless, and intolerant of not getting what they want. ADHD children have these characteristics to a marked degree. They are often, in a sense, extremes of the normal, as are very short or very tall people. Their characteristics are too much and too little of certain normal traits.

In families in which ADHD occurs on a temperamental basis, parents will frequently tell us that they had similar problems themselves when they were the age of their ADHD son or daughter. Being aware of this similarity can be useful or harmful, depending on the circumstances. It can be an advantage when the parents remember the problems they faced and the techniques that were most helpful in dealing with them. This may provide useful insight for helping the child. The awareness can be harmful when the parents play down the difficulties from ADHD. If the parents are unwilling to acknowledge that ADHD caused them difficulty (or still does), they may minimize the problems it is causing the child. If this happens, the parents may neglect serious problems that require recognition in order to be alleviated.

As scientists have studied ADHD children, they have begun to examine the psychological problems encountered among close relatives, particularly siblings and parents. They have observed two important factors. First, the siblings of ADHD children are more likely to have ADHD problems than are the siblings of children without ADHD. Second, as indicated above, the fathers and other close relatives of ADHD children report that they had such problems themselves as children (and, as we will see later, many probably have them as adults).

The psychiatrists who made these observations did not know at first whether the disorder was really hereditary or not. Perhaps parents who were psychologically disturbed brought up psychologically disturbed children. This would not be genetic, but would be a form of psychological heredity. Not everything that runs in families is genetic. And how strongly something runs in a family doesn't tell us if it is transmitted genetically or through learning. All the offspring of Chinese-speaking parents speak Chinese—this is 100 percent learned. A fairly small fraction of the children of a red-headed parent have red hair—and having red hair is a trait that is hereditarily transmitted. The problem is one of separating nature from nurture.

Investigators have tackled this problem in an ingenious way. First, they have studied ADHD in twins. Second, they have studied ADHD in adopted children and in children reared by foster parents. What they found from the twin studies is that in identical twins (those sharing the same genes) one twin is much more likely to have ADHD if the other one has it, but that in fraternal twins (those sharing genes no more similar than siblings would) one is no more likely to have ADHD than any brother or sister of the afflicted twin. The second studies, those of adopted and foster children, permit scientists to separate the influence of genetic factors from those of family upbringing. Those studies have found that (1) when raised in foster homes, full siblings of ADHD children are twice as likely as half siblings to have ADHD themselves; and (2) the biological parents of adopted-away ADHD children are more likely to have ADHD than the biological parents of adopted-away non-ADHD children. The implication is that the disorder is being transmitted genetically. There are also observations that suggest rearing factors do not play a primary role. Adopting parents of ADHD children have no more ADHD than the adopting parents of non-ADHD children. The same is not true of biological parents who rear their own ADHD children. They are much more likely than those adopting parents to have symptoms of full-fledged ADHD. The implication is that the problems they show in child-rearing are not only those encountered by any parents of an ADHD child but may sometimes be a sign of their own ADHD and not the cause of their child's.

Pieces of the puzzle continue to fall into place as scientists study the functioning of the brain and the makeup of our genes. With new techniques that allow us to picture the many structures within the brain, scientists are finding, for example, that some people with ADHD and learning disorders have brains shaped differently from those of people without these disorders. Other investigators have recently examined the genes of ADHD children and found some differences associated with ADHD. If confirmed by others, it will not only prove that a specific genetic abnormality plays a role in ADHD, but it will also mean that a blood test will eventually be able to help diagnose the condition.

Although these genetic findings suggest that certain types of parents are more likely to have ADHD children, the studies do not indicate that such parents will inevitably have them.

OTHER CAUSES OF ADHD

■

Although temperament and inheritance are far and away the most frequent causes of ADHD, physicians have investigated several other possible causes. The first is lead poisoning. It has been known for a long time that people who absorb too much lead develop both psychological and neurological (damage to nerves) problems. In fact, it was known forty years ago that some children who ate lead (usually in the form of lead paint on walls, windowsills, or cribs) developed ADHD. What has recently been discovered is that lead poisoning may have developed in children who never consumed lead. Studies in big cities have suggested that some children who were diagnosed as "hyperactive" had mild, chronic lead poisoning, resulting from breathing automobile fumes. As everyone probably knows, a chemical compound containing lead was long used in gasoline to improve the performance of cars. When the gasoline was burned, the lead heated, became a gas, and passed into the air. In large cities, it may have been sufficient merely to breathe the air to take in too much lead.

Other possible causes of ADHD have been proposed that relate to diet—specifically a diet that contains food additives or is high in sugar—and allergies. Some years ago a West Coast allergist (a physician specializing in the diagnosis and treatment of allergies) claimed that ADHD might be caused by the food children eat. These claims received serious attention from a number of scientific investigators, who conducted controlled experiments on the effect of food additives. In controlled experiments, the investigator makes allowances for people's expectation about a treatment. If people believe they are receiving a helpful treatment, they will often respond satisfactorily, even if their difficulties are physical and not mental. Thus, if ADHD children participate in an experiment that they—or their parents—believe will help them, they might function—or their parents might *think* the children function—better on the basis of that belief alone. Or, if an ADHD child perceives that a diet especially prepared *just for the child* brings him or her to the center of attention, that child's behavior might actually improve (perhaps temporarily).

As a control for such problems, investigators in one experiment used an innovative approach. They arranged with families of ADHD children to remove all food from the house. Each week the head of the household ordered the food the family would need for that week and the experimenters supplied all of it. With the permission of participating families, the experimenters sometimes included additives in the food and sometimes did not, but did not inform the families about those changes in the food. The investigators then examined the children's behavior both at home and in school. What they found is that the presence of food additives did not affect children to any appreciable degree. Their problems persisted when food additives were deleted, and their problems did not become worse when food additives were reinserted.

In other studies two food additives have been reported to produce behavioral effects in some children. One author reported on a child whose behavior was considerably worsened when he (without awareness) received aspartame, an artificial sweetener, as opposed to how he responded when given sugar. However this *one* child responded, aspartame has not been shown to systematically worsen the behavior of *groups* of ADHD children. The wisest course to follow is to use aspartame with moderation, particularly in younger children. In another study, investigators found that in a group of "hyperactive" children a little more than 10 percent showed improvement in their behavior when they were placed on a diet free of a particular food coloring, tartrazine. Their behavior worsened (they had more restlessness, irritability, and sleep problems) when tartrazine was reintroduced (without the children's or their parent's knowledge) into their diet. However, the investigators did *not* report a comparison between treating the children with medication and eliminating the dye from their diet. Eliminating the additive may have made some of the children better, but it did not necessarily make them well.

Many parents have been concerned whether sugar can cause the symptoms of ADHD. Scientific studies have found that sugar, a carbohydrate, cannot produce the symptoms of ADHD. ADHD children may *sometimes* respond to sugars in a way different from children without the disorder, but the effects are not marked. In one study ADHD children did better receiving carbohydrate than they did receiving protein! Two researchers have summarized: "Clearly, the maintenance of reasonable sugar intake in the presence of good nutrition and high protein intake is different than the exaggerated claims that sugar causes ADHD or that sugar-free diets are an effective treatment [for ADHD]."

What is true about sugar and ADHD is also true—in reverse order—about vitamins and ADHD. Just as too much sugar is not a cause of ADHD, a deficiency of vitamins is not a cause of ADHD. Attempts to improve the symptoms of ADHD by administering large doses of vitamins (and/or minerals) could in fact backfire, since large doses of some vitamins may be harmful.

Some allergists have claimed that allergies to natural foods may cause ADHD. Children with definite food allergies sometimes develop what is known as the tension-fatigue syndrome. In this condition, the child develops symptoms of excess fatigue (which may be accompanied by an increase in motor activity and restlessness), increased irritability, and a resulting increase in negative behavior. When the food allergy is appropriately treated—by eliminating the offending food from the diet—the child's behavior also improves. However, the behavior typical of the tension-fatigue syndrome bears only a superficial resemblance to ADHD. Though the child may be more restless and irritable, he doesn't have the other symptoms that go along with ADHD. If the child already had ADHD and in addition develops a food allergy with accompanying behavioral changes, this can be expected to make his ADHD much worse. If the food allergy is treated, the ADHD child's behavior should also improve, but his ADHD problems will remain. Thus, although food allergy may worsen ADHD in some cases, there is no evidence to suggest that allergies cause ADHD.

One study of children known to be allergic found that there was an improvement in ADHD symptoms when these children were placed on an elimination diet. The approach is to give the child those few foods that are known rarely to cause allergies and then, if the child benefits, to introduce new foods one at a time until behavioral problems reoccur. The food allergy-free diet may have made some of the ADHD children better, but did it make them *well*? Again, as with the tartrazine study, there is one important issue that this study did not investigate: a comparison between medication and an allergy-free diet.

Children with chronic hay fever also demonstrate behavioral changes when their hay fever is under poor control. They may become tired and irritable, with accompanying restlessness. Again, if the hay fever is successfully treated, their behavior often improves. Since hay fever is a common condition, many ADHD children can be expected to have this allergy in addition to their ADHD. If this is the case, treatment for the hay fever might be expected to help the child, but, again, it cannot be expected to eliminate completely his ADHD problems.

There is one cautionary point: placing a child on a special diet may also be unintentionally placing the child on a nutritionally poor diet. When food additive-free diets are given or when possible allergy-producing foods are eliminated, one must make sure that the diet contains a well-balanced mixture of carbohydrates, proteins, and fats. It is not enough to simply place a child (or an adult) on a diet and then supplement it with vitamins or minerals. Dietary treatment is not a treatment that a parent should try on his or her own. Either diet must be constructed and checked out by a physician or nutritionist. And again, if these diets make the child better, one must still find out whether or not they make the child well. To repeat: how important are additives and allergies in the production of ADHD? With the best information available, the answer appears to be that they are uncommon causes.

Another factor sometimes said to be a cause of ADHD is hypoglycemia, which is low blood sugar. To a physician, hypoglycemia is not present unless the blood sugar drops below a certain level, and if the blood sugar is under that level, it may indicate some underlying disease or disorder. Hypoglycemia defined in this way is a very uncommon condition. When the blood sugar does drop below a certain level, most people will have odd feelings, including light-headedness, a sense of weakness, irritability, a cold sweat, and palpitations. They often feel anxious. Only the irritability reminds one of the symptoms of ADHD.

Even though hypoglycemia is uncommon, its diagnosis is frequently made. In many cases this is a mistake. The over-diagnosis of hypoglycemia may happen because some people experience mild changes, like those previously described, when the blood sugar is low but still within the normal range. Some evidence suggests that experiencing these symptoms, even though the blood sugar is within normal range, occurs more frequently in people who are nervous or high-strung. Since ADHD children are frequently nervous and tense, that could explain why many people think that ADHD children may have hypoglycemia.

I have emphasized the importance of physiological contributions to Attention-Deficit Hyperactivity Disorder for two reasons. First, many people are unaware of them. Second, they are the most common causes of the problem. In a few instances, they play a minor role. The size of the physiological contribution can vary. In some children it is very large; no matter how the children are raised, problems will appear. In other children there are only slight physiological contributions. With these children, problems will be minor unless substantial family problems exist. In some instances one finds that the child has done reasonably well until serious family problems arose. Sometimes one cannot be sure of the origin of the child's difficulties since serious family tensions have been present at least since the time of the child's birth.

No matter how the ADHD child's problems arise, they frequently lead to typical difficulties within the family. Some psychiatrists and psychologists see the family's stresses as being a cause of the ADHD child's problems. Sometimes they are. Very often they are not, but are instead understandable reactions to the burden of the child's unpredictable and difficult behavior.

Children, like adults, respond to distress in terms of their type of personality. ADHD children react by being moody, naughty, and restless. All families, of course, want to solve their internal problems; in families with ADHD children, some resolution of such conflicts becomes even more important.

NATURE AND EFFECTS OF THE TEMPERAMENTAL PROBLEMS

In any given child it is impossible to say how much of his personality and behavior is due to temperament (nature) and how much is the result of his life experience (nurture). By the time he is six or seven his temperament has affected his behavior, which in turn has affected others around him, and their reactions in turn have affected him. For example, an aggressive child (not necessarily an ADHD child) will have bothered others, who in turn will have gotten angry, punished, and rejected him. The child feels rejected because he has been rejected (experience), but he has been rejected because he has been aggressive (temperament). Furthermore, a rejected child is more likely to feel frustrated and act aggressively. Temperament and experience snowball; they move in a vicious circle. We will soon discuss the sorts of vicious circles that ADHD children get into.

The central inborn temperamental differences in ADHD children often include the following characteristic problems: (1) inattentiveness and distractibility, (2) impulsivity (the inability to inhibit oneself—to say "no" to oneself and follow through, (3) restlessness, (4) demandingness, (5) academic underachievement, (6) hyperreactivity, (7) low tolerance for frustration, (8) temper outbursts, (9) bossiness and stubbornness, and (10) instability of mood—easily becoming depressed or excited. These traits are biologically caused. They are *not* caused by the child's upbringing. However, these inborn traits affect experience and can also be affected by experience. We will now discuss the ways in which this can happen.

SCHOOL BEHAVIOR

Although school problems were addressed in the previous chapter, they are so common and so important that it may be useful to explain again how they arise. To repeat: inattentiveness, distractibility, lack of stick-to-itiveness, and learning disorders (when present) interfere with academic progress despite the presence of a normal IQ. Even if the ADHD child does not have special learning difficulties, he will have a harder time learning than his intellectual peers will. To learn, a child must tolerate frustration. Some subjects are hard to understand and cannot be mastered without stick-to-itiveness. To learn, a child must pay attention. Intelligence is not enough. If the child cannot pay attention to what is being taught, he is, for all practical purposes, not there. To learn, a child must have patience. Elementary school requires a good deal of (boring) repetition, practice, and drill. A child who cannot force himself to complete tedious, disagreeable school tasks will have trouble in mastering reading, spelling, and arithmetic. The ADHD child is highly likely, therefore, to fall behind and become an underachiever. As the child gets further behind, he will experience more frustration and criticism from teachers, parents, and fellow students. His parents will nag him for not doing his homework. He may be placed in a catch-up class or a special learning disability class. He will regard himself as stupid and may be taunted as a "retard" by other children.

The problems of the ADHD child change as he becomes older and progresses into advanced grades. Entry into junior high school amplifies his problems for several reasons. First, junior high school is less structured. The ADHD child must monitor himself to be sure he goes where he is supposed to go at different times. Second, he has a number of different teachers. Because they know him less well than his elementary school teacher did, they are less likely to appreciate the possible strengths beneath his obvious weaknesses. Third, he begins to get homework that requires planning and application. No matter how smart he is, to be successful he must approach his homework systematically. In subjects requiring reading and outlining, he may be particularly handicapped. For all these reasons, if ADHD persists, academic problems typically increase in junior high school. These realistic problems combined with the special psychological problems some ADHD children develop in adolescence, along with the typical psychological problems that often affect non-ADHD adolescents, can make the early teens a very difficult period for the ADHD child.

Lack of success breeds low self-esteem and lack of enthusiasm. Even if the ADHD youngster outgrows his distractibility and inattentiveness, he may be so far behind and so soured on school that he only wants out. Although he may now be "normal" physiologically and although the temperamental problems may have diminished or disappeared, he is so scarred by school that he has acquired a marked distaste for it and may even drop out.

RELATIONSHIPS WITH OTHER CHILDREN

Because of his bossiness, his teasing, his "play it my way or not at all" attitude, some ADHD children are likely to be disliked by other children, and since they may not be very sensitive to the feelings of others they may constantly do the wrong things. (This applies only to those ADHD children who are bossy—some, not all.) Even if they are not bossy, other problems associated with ADHD may interfere with their peer relations. If the child is a boy and has coordination problems, the social problem will be worse. If he is chosen eighteenth when baseball teams are chosen, he will think little of himself. If, in addition, he has a temper tantrum when he strikes out, his popularity will not go up. In order to be liked he may resort to a number of maneuvers that will get him in trouble with both children and adults. He may boast, brag, lie, clown, or show off. As he gets older, he may try to prove his worth by doing the most dangerous, and most self-destructive, things: stealing, climbing to the highest place, and so forth. Note how the temperamental characteristics (demandingness, hyperactivity) lead to experience (rejection) that can lead to misguided attempts to improve relationships; the resultant social complications may reinforce the low self-esteem and make social interaction even more difficult.

In his relationships with his brothers and sisters, the same temperamental problems lead to other social difficulties. All brothers and sisters are jealous of one another from time to time. The ADHD child's behavior and the reactions that it produces in his parents predictably produce even more sibling envy and resentment than are common in any family. All the problems ordinarily associated with these sources of jealousies are aggravated and intensified. The ADHD child's brothers and sisters are probably favored because they are "good children" and he is "bad." They get more praise, he gets more blame, and he is jealous of them. On the other hand, he receives more attention than they do—because he both demands and requires it—and they may be jealous of him. Endless squabbling is often the result. Another, and unexpected, complication sometimes occurs if the ADHD child is treated and improves. The "good" children start showing problems! There are two explanations for this: first, they may previously have had problems but no one had noticed because the ADHD child's problems had been so much greater; second, the other children may have had no problems but have probably enjoyed their identification as the good children. When their ADHD brother or sister improves, they lose their enviable position and then manifest behavior that is very similar to the reactions of a child when a brother or sister is born. They may become jealous, act immaturely, and demand more attention. Fortunately, this does not always happen. I mention it only because it is upsetting when it occurs unexpectedly and is less upsetting when one knows that it can occur.

RELATIONSHIPS WITH PARENTS

The ADHD child's relationship with his parents is burdened by the difficulties encountered throughout his development. Because of his temperamental problems, the ADHD child often tends to be unsatisfiable from infancy. The mother cannot stop his colic, cannot handle his sleep disturbances, cannot satisfy him or make him happy. As he grows older, his hyperactivity, his impulsivity, and the other behavior problems I have discussed add tensions to family life. Nothing the parents seem to do helps very much or for very long. Probably the most common parental complaint is the difficulty in disciplining the ADHD child. The child is inattentive and rapidly forgets. He is told to clean his room, but when he is half-finished (or one-tenth finished), he starts doing something else. He is told not to jump down the stairs, stops for a while, and then impulsively does it again. He is not totally unresponsive to discipline. But he is much less responsive than non-ADHD children. If parents are very firm and very consistent, they will find that the ADHD child can be disciplined—at least to some extent. If they are not firm and not consistent, they may discover that he is almost totally out of control. How he is handled will often (not always) make a large difference. This is obviously of great importance in management and will be discussed in Chapter 5.

The difficulty in controlling the ADHD child's impulsivity has several disturbing effects. First, the child is a disappointment. Second, the child's chronic misbehavior is likely to make the parents angry. Third, the parents may see themselves as inept and inadequate. These feelings bring further emotional complications because the parents believe that they are not "supposed" to frequently feel angry toward their children. There are many emotions that people are not supposed to feel. One should not hate one's parents or one's child or envy one's sister. But such feelings do arise and, when they do, people tend to suppress them. They pretend they are not there, they ignore them, and they refuse to acknowledge them. Usually people are successful in these attempts and most of the time they are unaware that these feelings exist. Every now and then, however, in everyone, such feelings break through. When they do, one usually feels bad and guilty. When the parents of the ADHD child become aware of their angry feelings, they feel even more inadequate, and guilty and depressed as well. These feelings not only are highly distressing but also are likely to lead to techniques of child-rearing that aggravate the ADHD child's problems. Since reward and punishment seem ineffective in discipline, the parents are already confused, frustrated, and baffled. The anger the child engenders may make the parents act with excessive harshness. They may remove bicycle or TV privileges for a week. They may spank the child a little too hard. The parents' awareness of their severity (to a small child!) tends to produce further guilt, which leads them to try to atone by being more lenient. Frequently this leads to a pattern of alternating excessive discipline and excessive permissiveness, a pattern that is the opposite of the consistent atmosphere in which the child functions best. It may be that the child's behavior is making his parents behave inconsistently, or—and here is a further complication—since ADHD is genetically transmitted, the child may have one parent whose ADHD symptoms have not disappeared. If they have not, he has a parent who has been inconsistent, hot tempered, perhaps harsh, and likely unpredictable. This contrasts with the parent he needs: one who is consistent, even-tempered, tolerant, and predictable.

Severe and harsh discipline (which is very different from firm discipline) can produce certain kinds of "problems," or maladjusted behavior, in *any* child, and these responses sometimes appear in the ADHD child. Someone weak who feels he is being treated too harshly will feel resentful. But he has only limited ways of fighting back. He may comply resentfully, doing the job to the letter but not in the spirit of the law. He may merely pretend to comply. He may, at the risk of further punishment, dig in his heels and be negative, ornery, or stubborn. He may attempt to strike back by doing annoying, naughty, or hurtful things on another occasion. Nobody likes always being told what to do and what not to do. Even if the parent is a saint, the ADHD child (who finds it difficult to inhibit himself) will feel as if he is receiving more than his share of do's and don'ts and will be more inclined to stiffen his back in protest.

This friction leads to problems in other areas. As the parent-child problems multiply, the ADHD child will feel angry with his parents, but if one expresses anger at a loved one, one runs the risk of driving the loved one away. So in some cases the anger may not be expressed very directly. It can spill over and get taken out on a relatively innocent bystander, such as a playmate or teacher. This anger can also be completely bottled up. In adults this may be associated with psychosomatic disorders. For example, a person may keep his feelings inside himself and grow tense; in some instances the individual may actually get spasms and muscle pains (as expressed in the phrase "you give me a pain in the neck"). Lastly, the anger may be taken out on the child. This phenomenon is most surprising from the commonsense point of view, but is frequently seen in very angry and inhibited adults. They will have accidents and hurt themselves; they will engage in behavior that results in humiliation or punishment. The same kind of behavior can sometimes be seen in the ADHD child.

To further compound and complete the difficulties, the child's behavior often causes disagreement and dispute between the parents. Both parents perceive the child as behaving poorly, and each tends to blame the other for disciplining or treating the child inadequately. In particular, the father is apt to notice that he is more effective in controlling the child. He is, of course, less frequently around the home, and when he appears he is likely to lower the boom, with the result that the child heaves to, at least briefly. The father's natural remark to his wife is: "I can control him—why can't you?" His wife, who spends much more time with the child, replies, "You can't treat him like that all day long," and the fight begins. Many parents have different views on how much strictness and severity are necessary in discipline. A parent whose own experience as a child has been with harsh discipline tends to favor this approach, and one whose experience has been gentler is likely to oppose it. Consequently, one sometimes sees the formation of family triangles. One parent will be cast in the role of the child's defender while the other becomes the prosecutor. The prosecutor parent, who is the odd man out, then has an additional problem. Not only does he (or she) have a difficult child, but also his (or her) spouse is siding with the child against him. The parent who has been pushed out then feels jealous of his own child. Again, jealousy is one of those feelings that parents are not "supposed" to have, but do. Brief reflection about one's own family or the families of friends should quickly bring to mind numerous illustrations of the complications, animosities, and guilt that can ensue.

Another and almost universal familial complication exists. In the recent past almost all child psychiatrists and psychologists have maintained that most of the behavioral problems seen in children were the results of the manner in which they were raised by their parents. Most parents who have done any reading on child-rearing are aware of these notions but do not realize that they are becoming very much out of date. Such parents reach what they think is an obvious conclusion. They have a child with behavior difficulties. Children's behavior difficulties are the results of their parents' difficulties. Therefore, the parents—they themselves—must be either stupid or evil. Their child's difficulties are not only a serious problem for their offspring but are also a reflection of the parents' failure as parents. Unfortunately, many mental health workers may reinforce the parents in this view. There are still a few (and a decreasing number of) psychiatrists, psychologists, social workers, teachers, and school guidance counselors who are unaware of the evidence for the physical basis of ADHD. They, too, believe that the child's problems are a reflection of his parents' problems. They will inform the parents, subtly or otherwise, that they are responsible for their child's difficulties. This will either intensify the parents' sense of guilt, anxiety, and depression, or lead them to deny that there is anything wrong with the child. The latter course would be difficult to follow, but rather than be labeled as bad parents of a bad child, some people will deny the evidence of their senses and proclaim that their child is perfectly normal but misunderstood by others. This is an understandable, common, and unfortunate technique that delays or prevents the problem from being solved. Many parents of ADHD children have accused themselves for many years, and a final prosecution by experts may lead them to defend themselves by denying the existence of problems in the child, which in turn leads to the child's not receiving treatment. Contrary to usual belief, family disturbances are often the result and not the cause of a child's problems.

Certainly, these parent-child relationship patterns are not seen in all families with ADHD children, and not even in most of them. They have been presented to illustrate how temperament in the child can produce changes in those around him, which in turn will produce psychological changes in the child. Notice that the temperament of the parent is very important in this equation. If the parent is hot tempered or impulsive because of either temperament or experience, he or she is more likely to become involved with and intensify the child's problems. Parents of ADHD children need to pay a great deal of attention to detail, must keep themselves from overreacting, must not let feelings of frustration, disappointment, or anger influence the child, and should be unusually well organized.

THE CHILD'S FEELINGS ABOUT HIMSELF

Although the ADHD child sometimes feels anger in response to his parents' reactions to his behavior, he more often has other reactive feelings that are more self-destructive. Because the child is rejected, criticized, and told he is exasperating, he will feel unlovable and unworthy and think little of himself. His teachers are likely to say such things as, "You are bright enough to do better. Why don't you try harder? . . .

You could do better if you cared" (adding "like your brother or sister"—if they attended the same school). He is unpopular with his peers. They choose him less for games or not at all. He is not invited to parties or sleepovers. Because he is unpopular and highly reactive to teasing, he is frequently teased. His parents are usually exasperated. They continually express their annoyance, anger, or disappointment with him. Even if they do not openly compare him with his brothers and sisters, he can see that his parents like his siblings better. Parental self-control can diminish these feelings, but it cannot prevent them. Even though he is somewhat thick-skinned and even though people may say nothing, the child cannot help noticing how people react to him.

Our self-esteem is formed on the basis of others' responses to us. We learn that we are attractive, nice, or bright, depending on whether others consider us good-looking, pleasant, and intelligent. The ADHD child has a low opinion of himself. This is not neurotic, it is rational. He is failing at school, with his peers, and with his parents. He fails in all the important areas of a child's life. He feels he is dumb, lazy, disobedient, and unlikable because that is the way his world regards him.

Obviously, anything that can help the child change his behavior will prevent him from suffering the consequences of that behavior. Although a child may eventually outgrow the physiological and the temperamental problems, the psychological difficulties he has had because of the temperamental problems may persist. He will have learned—and not forgotten—patterns of psychological maladjustment. On the other hand, if the physiological problems and symptoms can be kept in check until he outgrows them, he will avoid many bad experiences and grow up more easily. He will do better in school and enjoy better relationships with his family and friends. He will not suffer severe consequences from his attention-deficit hyperactivity disorder. Many ADHD children can now be helped to achieve this major goal, as we will see in Chapter 5.

4

The Development of the Child
with Attention-Deficit
Hyperactivity Disorder

■

In Chapter 2 on the characteristics of the ADHD child, I discussed the problems a child with ADHD encounters, and how these change as he grows. I also mentioned that the sequence of problems is not inevitable, and that may cause ADHD children to grow out of their problems as they become older. An obvious and reasonable question that parents might ask is what the fate of their ADHD child will be. Ten years ago we did not know. As I will explain, this question is now easier to answer.

Because of new clinical data, we are obtaining a picture of the changes in the condition over time. The information comes from two sources. The first consists of studies of ADHD children who were followed from childhood into adolescence. We are beginning to obtain information about the adult outcome of ADHD children from a second source—two scientific studies, started about fifteen years ago, that systematically followed and compared a group of ADHD children with a group of non-ADHD children and evaluated them into their mid-twenties. These two studies, one conducted in New York City and the other in Montreal, are described later in this chapter.

Physicians who have treated "hyperactive" children over a period of years have repeatedly noted that in some of the children the problems tend to change, become less severe, and disappear with age. This sort of progress caused some physicians to label ADHD a developmental lag. (The implication is that the ADHD child, who is immature, is like a child who is unusually short for his age. Both are likely to catch up, to become mature or taller, but later than most children.) In many ADHD children some of the more troublesome symptoms gradually diminish and finally disappear around the time of puberty; in some children such improvements may occur earlier and in some later. However, recent studies indicate that 70 to 80 percent of ADHD children will not outgrow their symptoms in adolescence and will have continuing problems in school, with their families, and with their peers. In all ADHD children some symptoms change and disappear. The ADHD child may wet his bed longer than the child without ADHD, but he does not wet his bed forever. Similarly, restlessness and fidgetiness may diminish with age. However—and this is extremely important—even though these symptoms may vanish, other ADHD symptoms may persist. Difficulty in concentrating, lack of stick-to-itiveness, and impulsivity may remain. Obvious hyperactivity may have disappeared whereas many of the other problems lingered for several years. Many adults continue to have ADHD-related problems. The practical consequence is that treatment, when effective, may need to be continued for several years after the most obvious and distressing symptoms have vanished.

In considering the practical implications of the development of the ADHD child, one must ask this question: "Is the persistence of symptoms due to the persistence of the temperamental (biochemical) problem, or is it due to maladjusted patterns of behavior that were learned because of the (no longer existing) temperamental problem?" The question cannot be answered in a general way, but a sensitive clinician can often give an approximate answer for an individual child. In some children, the problems do seem to persist because of the persisting temperamental difficulty. In other children, the persistence of symptoms seems to be the result of behavior that was learned and now remains, so to speak, as a habit. (Similarly, a child who had broken his right arm and learned to write with his left hand might well retain indefinitely the ability to write with his left hand even after the fracture healed.) Some persisting symptoms were originally considered psychological but now seem of physiological origin. For example, when adults in their thirties and forties with ADHD symptoms are given drug treatment for the first time and it is effective, they usually demonstrate greatly improved attention span, increased organizational abilities, and substantial improvement in several other areas that will be discussed in Chapter 6 (accompanied by an increase in self-esteem). Medication changes brain chemistry; it does not correct inadequate learning. The implication of this observation is that the persisting organizational problems were the result of abnormal brain chemistry, not the inadequate *learning* of organizational skills.

The temperamental difficulty often responds well to medical treatment. This will be discussed in the next chapter. Some behavior is learned better and embedded more deeply if it is learned when young and is harder to change when older. If the immigrant learns a second language when he is ten or twelve, he may always speak it with the accent of his first learned, native tongue. If children are exposed to a foreign language before they are five or six, they learn it more easily and remember more of it than does an intelligent adult, and speak it without an accent. Habits and attitudes, like skills, are learned more quickly and better when young, and habits learned when young are harder to unlearn. Further, some personality traits and attitudes developed in adolescence can be very durable, so it is desirable that the child have every physical and psychological advantage as he approaches that period. For example, in one study thin women who had been fat in childhood or adolescence were asked how they regarded themselves. Interestingly, only those women who had been fat in adolescence had suffered psychological effects and continued to regard themselves as unattractive, despite the fact that they were thin adults. Attitudes learned during the teenage years had stuck with them. The relevance for ADHD children is, I hope, obvious. The sooner that maladaptive learning can be prevented the better, for the child will have less difficulty in adolescence and later life than he would have otherwise. If such habits or attitudes are learned, the outlook is not grim. Learned habits can be unlearned, skills can be acquired, and new experiences can change personality throughout one's life. Chapter 5 will consider some psychological approaches that are pertinent here. But from what we know about children's growth and development, *early treatment would seem to be more effective than later treatment.*

When ADHD symptoms persist to a significant degree into adolescence, special issues arise because the ADHD problems interact with normal psychological changes that occur when a child is undergoing adolescence. From school age on, children's peers play an increasingly large role in their social development. As children enter adolescence, the impact of their friends becomes even greater. Distraught parents are frequently aware that their adolescent child adopts values of his peer group that are in opposition to previously accepted home values. The adolescent is strongly motivated to form close relationships with his peers. Intimacy with equals replaces intimacy with parents. Adolescents confide in each other, but often mumble or are mute with their parents.

Forming relationships with peers is sometimes a problem for the preadolescent ADHD child. For the ADHD adolescent who continues to lack social perceptiveness and interpersonal skills, problems with peers continue. If his ADHD handicaps affect the kinds of talents that make adolescents popular—for example, if he is poorly coordinated in athletic performance—he is additionally limited in making close friends. The lack of peer acceptance in adolescence is even more painful than it is in childhood.

Some ADHD children seem to get less pleasure from the activities that other children enjoy. They may require excitement and dangerous situations to experience the pleasure that other children derive from less stimulating activities. The search for excitement increases the possibility that the ADHD adolescent may associate with delinquent peers. A tendency toward depression (both in reaction to difficulties resulting from ADHD and perhaps as part of the ADHD itself) may also play a role in excitement seeking. The combination of continuing low self-esteem (amplified by peer rejection), impaired social skills, and impulsivity may lead the child to associate with any group of peers who accepts him, including those engaged in delinquent activities.

One of the major areas of psychological growth in adolescents is development of autonomy—feelings of self-sufficiency and freedom from one's parents. This is a healthy pattern, even if it causes temporary conflict between parents and adolescent. The severity of the conflict may depend on how the adolescent expresses increasing autonomy. Preferences for current adolescent fashions in music, hair styles, and clothing may produce mild parental irritation, but idealistic or activist political positions at variance with parental ones, or becoming a member of a social outgroup, can result in serious disruption of family bonds.

Another important adolescent developmental task is establishing relationships with the opposite sex, which requires social ease and social skills. Because of his social obtuseness, the ADHD adolescent may not be shy, but because of his social ineptitude, he stands a good chance of being unsuccessful.

Still another area—most conspicuous in those who showed insufficient conscience as children—is continuing problems with self-control. Self-control involves a number of psychological attributes that ADHD adolescents tend to be deficient in: control of impulsivity, empathy, and ability to perceive one's effect on others. These deficits are characterisitic of social immaturity and increase the possibility that the ADHD adolescent will become involved in delinquent acts. And indeed, systematic studies have shown that in adolescence formerly ADHD children *are* much more likely than their non-ADHD peers to develop alcohol and substance abuse and become involved in delinquent behavior. These studies are of *untreated* ADHD adolescents and may have included those with undiagnosed Conduct Disorder who are chronic rule-breakers.

The two systematic studies referred to earlier, one conducted in New York City and the other in Montreal, shed important light on the development of the ADHD child. In the New York City study, children first seen between the ages of six and twelve were reinterviewed at an average age of eighteen and then again at twenty-six. Investigators found that at age eighteen, 40 percent of the original ADHD children continued to have major problems, while at age twenty-six the number was about 10 percent. Two additional important findings were that, at ages eighteen and twenty-six, the ADHD children were much more likely to have problems with conduct (Oppositional Defiant Disorder and the more severe Conduct Disorder) and substance abuse. These figures may underestimate the persistence of the childrens' problems. The investigators based their diagnoses only on the childrens' report of symptoms; they did not interview their parents. We know that ADHD children at all ages—as well as ADHD adults—underestimate the extent and seriousness of their problems. When we interview adults with possible ADHD parents—and the adults' partners—we find that a much higher proportion are reported to have problems than the patients report themselves. This probably represents a serious understatement because they did not interview parents or other informants, and we know from our clinical work with ADHD adults that many patients see their ADHD problems as mild or minor; their partners see them as having moderate to severe problems.

The Montreal study also began with ADHD children between the ages of six and twelve. When reinterviewed fifteen years later, 66 percent of these children reported at least one symptom of restlessness, distractibility, or impulsivity as compared to about 5 percent in the group who had been normal children. About 20 percent had more severe problems, including—as in the New York City study—Conduct Disorders.

The relationship between ADHD and substance abuse in adult life is not clear. A number of studies of alcoholics have suggested that ADHD children may be likely not only to abuse alcohol but other substances. However, some of these studies did not separate children with "pure" ADHD from those with mixed ADHD and Conduct Disorders. It may be the mixed ADHD/conduct-disordered children who are more likely to abuse alcohol. From a practical standpoint, about one-quarter of ADHD children have an alcoholic parent.

There is one extremely important feature of the New York City and Montreal studies to keep in mind. The children participating in the research *did not continue* to receive treatment with medication, counseling, or remedial education. These studies tell us only what will happen if we do not provide continuing treatment to ADHD children. So what are the conclusions? They are three. First, based on the Montreal study ADHD probably continues to cause definite problems in adult life in one-third or more of instances. Another third will continue to have some ADHD symptoms that are not as prominent. Second, ADHD children, particularly if they have Oppositional Defiant Disorder, are much more likely than normal children to develop Conduct Disorder. Third, ADHD children, possibly only if they have Conduct Disorder as well, are probably more likely to develop alcohol and other substance abuse disorders.

These conclusions may be disheartening. However, early

and well-administered medical treatment, in combination with well-managed psychological treatment, may prevent—or greatly reduce—the psychological symptoms that develop on the basis of the physiological abnormalities. Such treatment, of course, does not cure the underlying physiological abnormalities, and perhaps the reason that some treatment programs in the past proved ineffective may simply be that they did not continue to administer medication as long as ADHD symptoms persisted. Without treatment, the number of children who continue to have problems is larger than was previously believed. Since we now have evidence that many ADHD children still have the same physiological difficulties in adult life (inattentiveness, hot temper, not being able to complete tasks, and so on) and continue to respond to medication, it seems obvious that some ADHD children may benefit from—and may need to take—medicine for many years after childhood. An area of high priority now being investigated is to determine if medication in addition to parent education, behavior therapy, and group therapy for children affects the "natural history" of ADHD. Can such treatment prevent ADHD problems later or enable the children to deal with them more effectively?

Recently, I and my colleagues and others who are doing research in ADHD have discovered that in a fairly large number of instances, ADHD problems persist into the thirties, forties, and fifties. And during the last few years, recognition of ADHD in adults has exploded (and, probably, sometimes been *overdiagnosed*). We first became aware of ADHD in adults in talking to the parents of ADHD children. Frequently, the parents mentioned that they had been inattentive and hyperactive in childhood, and many reported that some of their problems had become less severe with age but still bothered them to an annoying degree. These adults differed from ADHD children not only in that some of the problems were less severe than they had been, but also in that they had developed adult ways of coping with them. Of particular interest—and practical importance—was our discovery that many of the adults who continued to suffer from ADHD problems could benefit from treatment with medications as much as ADHD children.

Similarly, Learning Disorders may persist well into the thirties and forties. Although *apparently* (there is no really substantial information) spurts *may* occur at around age eight and in the early teens, during which Learning Disorders improve, there is an overall tendency for learning-disordered children to fall further and further behind with age. A large fraction of learning-disordered children continue to have serious problems well into adult life. In others, some improvement occurs, but learning-disordered children often continue to be slow readers and poor spellers, and if they have had difficulty with arithmetic, they continue to have problems in performing mathematical calculations.

How can we best summarize the findings to date? How frequently does ADHD persist into adult life? The crude estimate seems to be between one-third and two-thirds. The severity varies considerably, from those having mild symptoms of inattentiveness and disorganization—and perhaps restlessness—to those with a persistence of childhood symptoms that may have changed their form with maturity. The exact nature of these persisting symptoms will be discussed in Chapter 6, Attention-Deficit Hyperactivity Disorder in the Adult. However, the proportion of adults who have mild, moderate, or severe symptoms remains to be discovered.

5

Treatment of the Child with Attention-Deficit Hyperactivity Disorder

■

The treatment of the ADHD child can often be relatively straightforward. Because medication is of the greatest importance, treatment almost always requires the services of a physician. Nonmedical specialists, such as psychologists, educators, and social workers, may provide useful and sometimes absolutely necessary assistance, but they cannot assume primary responsibility for treatment. Since they are not trained to use and cannot prescribe medications, they are unable to supply the treatment that is both the best and sometimes the only one required. This must be emphasized because too often the ADHD child or his family is referred to a psychologist, social worker, or school guidance counselor. Such referrals are made because of psychological maladjustment in the child, problems in the family, or failure in school. These problems, as I have said, may be a result of ADHD in the child, and they may also worsen ADHD in the child. Family problems, which may prompt the family to seek help, may actually be the result of the ADHD child and may resolve themselves once treatment begins.

What sometimes happens is that the ADHD child is misdiagnosed and referred for help, and it is then noticed that his parents have marital problems. Someone then assumes that the child's problems are the result of family problems, and the parents receive treatment. This occurs frequently because the traditional view in child psychiatry had been that most children's problems are the product of their parents' or their families' problems. The difficulty is that a large number of married couples have serious problems. An increasingly large proportion of all marriages end in divorce. Of those that do not, perhaps half have serious difficulties. Thus, the chances are great that the parents of any child are having difficulties. If one looked at the parents of children with rheumatic fever, epilepsy, or mental retardation, one would find that a large number had marital problems. (And, in fact, some of these problems might be caused by the child's illness.) No one would expect that helping the parents would cure a child's rheumatic fever, epilepsy, or mental retardation. Helping the parents might, and probably would, make the child happier. Similarly, it is quite possible that the parents of an ADHD child are having marital difficulties; if one helps only the parents, the child will probably be more comfortable in some ways, but his basic problems will remain untouched and unchanged. Finally, since ADHD is frequently hereditary, the parent may have ADHD and the ADHD parent's own symptoms (such as being hot tempered or disorganized or impulsive) may make it hard for this parent to raise an ADHD child. Treatment of ADHD—or any other psychiatric disorder—in the parent will obviously be of great assistance in enabling the parent to carry out the psychological and behavioral management of the child. A major difficulty for the ADHD child is that his problems are sometimes not recognized as medical. His medical problems manifest themselves in his behavior and, until recently, all such problems were thought to be psychologically caused. The reasoning has been that if he, and perhaps his parents, has psychological problems, only psychological treatment is required because the behavioral problems, as we have emphasized, stem from biological differences. Normal children may have disturbed parents. Disturbed children may have normal parents. And disturbed children may have disturbed parents—and even here, the two sets of disturbances may be largely separate.

Almost all ADHD children have psychological problems. And some of these problems can be helped by psychological therapies. But as long as the temperamental problems remain, the psychological problems will continue to spring up. In other words, the young ADHD child—and the adolescent child in whom temperamental problems remain—will require treatment for those temperamental problems first. Psychotherapy may still be necessary and may benefit the child—and later I will discuss how—but unless his medical treatment is continued, it is almost certain that the original problems will recur.

Finally, the same principles hold for educational treatment. The school counselor will see the child with educational problems or behavioral problems or both. The counselor may assume that the behavioral problems are causing the academic ones, or that the academic problems are causing the behavioral problems. And the counselor is probably *partly* right in either case. The catch is that both kinds of problems can be separately caused by ADHD. Dealing with either without treating the underlying disorder may be helpful but it is not the best treatment.

To repeat: the help provided by trained professionals other than physicians can be important and sometimes necessary to the ADHD child and his family, but most ADHD children require medical treatment; at present only physicians are in a position to provide such treatment. Once the child has embarked on the basic course of medical treatment, it will be easier to decide whether the parents should also seek help for him from a psychologist, social worker, or teacher.

All three major forms of treatment are discussed in this chapter: medical, psychological, and educational. I will also add a few words about help for the youngster whose ADHD is discovered in adolescence.

MEDICAL TREATMENT

■

A very large fraction of ADHD children can be helped, often to a marked degree, by treatment with medication. In some children this may be the *only* treatment that is required. In others psychological and educational interventions may also be necessary. It is often difficult beforehand to determine how much of a child's trouble is caused by family difficulties and how much by his own temperament. Often, after a child has been treated with medications some of the problems may disappear while others will remain. The physician may then suggest psychological treatment for the family and the child, and/or educational intervention for the child.

The use of medication to treat children is sometimes upsetting to parents. Parents are troubled for various reasons and it may be useful to discuss them.

First, many parents have difficulty coming to terms with the fact that their child's behavior problems have a physical rather than a psychological basis; often this is because they find physical problems frightening. They may believe that in the area of behavior what is psychological can easily be remedied whereas what is physical cannot. They feel that a temper tantrum is soon over, but the chemically abnormal brain may never recover. For this reason they would rather believe that the problem is psychological. If the child's misbehavior is psychological, surely the powerful psychiatrists can change it, but how could his brain be cured? On both counts, the parents' information is incomplete. Fortunately, just as with many other serious physical problems, behavior malfunctions with physical origins can sometimes be easily remedied. On the other hand, psychological treatment is not always as effective as it is believed to be. Certain common forms of brain tumor that cause profound psychological disturbances can be easily removed, whereas, in contrast, some neuroses of psychological origin cannot be cured despite years of expensive and time-consuming psychological treatment. Pneumonia can often be cured with a single shot of penicillin. Pernicious anemia, formerly a fatal disease, can be completely cured by vitamin administration. But a child who has been neglected or physically, sexually, and psychologically abused during early childhood may never function normally, even if he later receives warm, considerate parental care and psychotherapy.

A second reason parents sometimes object to treatment with medication is that such treatment seems artificial. To many parents it does not appear to be a good way to get to the root of the problem. That may be so if the root of the problem is psychological, but in the case of ADHD it is generally physical. Because some regulatory functions of the brain are operating less efficiently than usual, chemical means must be used to improve their functioning. Medication can be regarded as a form of replacement therapy; that is, it apparently supplies chemicals that are lacking or causes the body to create more of the missing chemicals. At present, we can give no chemical that will permanently cure the deficiency. Unlike pneumonia, ADHD has no one-shot cure. Medication is necessary unless and until the brain, through its own growth and development, begins producing adequate amounts of the required chemicals. This is very similar to the treatment required for pernicious anemia, except that pernicious anemia requires administration of vitamin B_{12} throughout the patient's life; unlike the patient with pernicious anemia, the ADHD child may outgrow his difficulties.

A third reason parents sometimes object to medication is that they fear the child will become dependent on it. By dependency, parents generally mean two things. First, they fear that the medication is a substance currently feared as a drug of abuse. They sometimes worry that, like the drug addict, the child will feel so good after taking the medication that he will become addicted to it. This is never true of the medications employed by physicians in the treatment of ADHD. Children may be happy about the improvement in their lives that medicine helps to produce, but they never like the medicine. They do not get high from it. They don't get kicks from it. Medically, any nonnaturally occurring substance that is administered to a person with the hope of therapeutic results is a drug. Aspirin is a drug. So is penicillin. Certain forms of hormones are drugs. The problem is not whether a substance is called a medication or a drug but whether it is beneficial or harmful. As will be seen, most of the medications used in the treatment of ADHD are beneficial and carry very little risk.

A second form of dependency that parents sometimes fear is the need for the continuing use of medication to handle problems. In this respect the parents are correct, but this type of dependency is preferable to the ailment. Many ADHD children *do* need medicine to control their problem. The ADHD child is in a position similar to but less threatening than that of the child with diabetes, epilepsy, or rheumatic fever. Children with those disorders must take insulin, anti-epileptic drugs, or penicillin for the rest of their lives. The ADHD child may be luckier. Since many ADHD children may outgrow their major symptoms, the ADHD child may have to take medication for only a part of his life.

In discussing the major medications employed by most physicians in the treatment of ADHD children, their effects, and their administration, my aim will be to help the parent understand the physician's treatment goals. I will not be presenting an exhaustive list of medications, and of course this discussion is not intended to enable parents to treat their child by themselves. Parents who are aware of how a drug should act, what side effects it can produce, and what (if any) possible hazards accompany its use are in a much better position to assist their physicians in the treatment of their child. With this in mind, let us now turn to some general aspects of the administration of medication to ADHD children.

The first very important point to be made is that several medications are potentially helpful for children with ADHD. It is impossible to predict how a child will respond to a particular medication. Some children respond well to one medication and not to another. It may be necessary to try several before the best one can be found.

Another important principle to keep in mind is that, at beginning any course of medication, a physician will start at the smallest dose that is ever effective, since he or she does not wish to give more medication than is necessary. Because of this, it is often necessary to increase the amount of medicine considerably. This should be no cause for alarm. Children differ greatly, and some children need much larger amounts of medication than others. The amount of medication is not necessarily related to the seriousness of the problem. For example, some ADHD children with extreme symptoms may require only very small amounts of medicine while those whose symptoms are much less severe may need larger amounts.

Many medications produce side effects. A side effect is an undesired by-product of the administration of medicine. For example, aspirin sometimes produces irritation of the lining of the stomach and mild abdominal pain. Antihistamines, given for hay fever, sometimes cause sleepiness. The medications used in treating ADHD children will sometimes produce side effects. When I discuss the individual medications, I will mention these side effects.

Lastly, all medicines (including aspirin and penicillin) may produce allergic reactions. An allergic reaction occurs only in a small proportion of people who receive medication. Some medications are much more likely to produce allergies than others. The drugs most commonly used in treating ADHD children, the stimulant drugs, very rarely produce allergies. Some medications that are used when the stimulant drugs do not seem to be the best treatment for an individual child are somewhat more likely to produce allergies. Parents should know the symptoms of allergies and should contact the doctor if they do occur. Although this rarely happens, if allergies are allowed to go on, they sometimes become worse. Some major symptoms are quite obvious: skin rash and hives. One other major symptom that many people are not aware of is a decrease in white blood cell count, which results in an increased susceptibility to infections. When such an allergy occurs it is most common for a person to develop a sore throat and a high fever. Of course, most children who are not receiving medications of any sort occasionally get sore throats and high fevers, but a physician should immediately see a child who is receiving medication and develops such symptoms.

STIMULANT DRUGS

The medications most frequently used in the treatment of ADHD children are the stimulant drugs. The most common are Dexedrine and Desoxyn, which are amphetamines, and Ritalin (methylphenidate). The amphetamines were introduced in the late 1930s. Ritalin was first synthesized in 1955 and began to be used in the early 1970s. Cyclert (pemoline) is another stimulant drug that is also widely used. A fourth stimulant, Adderall, has been introduced recently. It is a combination of two amphetamines and its dose is thought by some to last for a longer time than Dexedrine and Desoxyn. This would certainly be useful, but there is no firm confirmation about this. Two-thirds or more of ADHD children respond well to one of these drugs. Although the drugs are about equal in effectiveness, a particular child may respond better to one than to another. If one drug provides only moderate improvement or produces annoying side effects, a physician may try a different drug.

A less commonly used stimulant drug, Cylert (generic name: pemoline) has been generally employed as a "second-line drug" (meaning only if the first-choice drug was not effective). It is being less frequently used since the manufacturer reported that as of 1996 there had been at least thirteen cases of acute liver failure and eleven deaths in patients taking Cylert. This safety record has to be compared with those of Dexedrine, Desoxyn, and Ritalin, which have been found to have remarkably few side effects, have been administered to many, many more patients than Cylert, and have never been reported to produce such toxicity. It is to be expected that physicians will either discontinue the use of Cylert or use it only with extreme precautions, and in very special instances. Cylert has been withdrawn from the market in Canada.

Despite their effectiveness and safety, amphetamines and methylphenidate have acquired a bad reputation because they may cause adults to become high and psychologically dependent on them. (Amphetamine is well known as "speed.") Cylert does not appear to have this property, and little or no abuse has occurred. (This was considered a desirable property since it could be used to treat substance-abusing patients who had ADHD.) Stimulant drugs have a much different effect in ADHD children than they do in normal adults. Instead of becoming high or excited, these drugs in general calm down ADHD children and sometimes (rarely) they may even become somewhat sad. Children do not become addicted to these medications; there is absolutely no danger that this will occur. If the ADHD child's problems persist into adolescence, many physicians will discontinue the use of the stimulant drugs and substitute medications that are not habit-forming in adults. However, many physicians who have treated numerous ADHD children may continue to use the stimulant drugs well into adolescence—with caution—because of their medical impression that these children do not begin to respond to the drugs as normal adults do unless they have outgrown their ADHD problems. This remains only an impression because we have no hard data on how children who have outgrown their ADHD resond to stimulants.

The hundreds of ADHD adults I have studied have generally shown the same response to medication as ADHD children. They become calm rather than excited, and they do not get high. Furthermore, taking notice of the fact that adults weigh more than children and therefore may need proportionately larger doses, the ADHD adults I have treated continue to benefit from the same relatively small doses, correcting for weight. This contrasts with adults who abuse stimulant drugs for their euphoric effects, who must escalate the dosage, sometimes to ten times or more, to continue to receive the drug effect.

Effectiveness

When the stimulant drugs are effective, they improve many symptoms of the syndrome. ADHD children generally (1) become calmer and less active; (2) develop a longer span of attention; (3) become less stubborn and easier to manage (they "mind" better); (4) are often more sensitive to the needs of others and much more responsive to discipline and the wishes of others; (5) have longer fuses and fewer or no temper tantrums; (6) experience fewer emotional ups and downs; (7) show a decrease in impulsivity, waiting before they act, and may begin to plan ahead; (8) demonstrate an improvement in school performance (listening, following instructions, completing tasks, getting better grades; (9) improve their handwriting; and (10) become less disorganized. When stimulants work, the child matures and may function better—at least temporarily—than he ever has in his life. The response of the

ADHD child to stimulant medication is unlike that to any other medication in psychiatry. At best, most other treatments restore a patient to his previous level of functioning. The temporary psychological growth that occurs when stimulants are effective is very different from simple slowing down or quieting. And it is a very different effect from what the parent—if he does not have ADHD—may have experienced with tranquilizers or stimulants. When used by normal adults, tranquilizers produce a relaxing effect and stimulants an exciting effect. Neither drug stabilizes mood, cools tempers, makes one more law-abiding, dampens impulsivity, or helps one to plan ahead.

The widespread effect of stimulant medication on various psychological functions has led child psychiatrists to believe that the brain chemistry of people with ADHD is in some ways different from that of others. The medication seems to compensate at a basic level for this chemical difference, affecting behavior in many diverse areas. It should be emphasized that these effects are very different from those of the so-called tranquilizing drugs. Tranquilizing drugs may slow a child down, but they do not increase his attention span, personal sensitivity, or reasonableness.

If the child is responsive to amphetamines and methylphenidate, the medications are usually effective immediately. In a few instances, the effects described may take as long as a week or two to appear. The effects of pemoline are seen much more slowly; it may take two or three weeks for pemoline's full benefit to be realized.

Dosage

Parents' evaluation of their child's adjustment will play an important role in the doctor's decision to increase or decrease the dose of the medication. The parents should know something about the dosages ordinarily employed. Medications are usually measured in milligrams. A milligram (one-thousandth of a gram) is a unit of weight, about 1/30,000th of an ounce. The amount of the amphetamines Dexedrine Desoxyn, or Adderall an ADHD child may require usually ranges from about 10 to 60 milligrams a day. Ritalin (methylphenidate) is only half as potent, so the amount required can range from 20 to 120 milligrams a day. Occasionally there are exceptions in either direction: a very few children will require less than these dosages, and a few will require more. Overall, about as many children respond to the amphetamines as they do to methylphenidate. However, any individual child may respond better to one or the other. If the response is good but not complete to one of the amphetamines, then Ritalin may be tried, and if the response to Ritalin is good but not complete, then the amphetamines may be tried. An additional concern is how frequently medication must be given. This involves the availability of long-acting formulations. Unfortunately, the current long-acting form's release of medication is not ideal. The capsules or tablets may release too much medication initially, followed by too low a dose thereafter. These problems are discussed below.

Dexedrine is available in two forms: 5-milligram tablets and 5-, 10-, and 15-milligram long-acting capsules (Dexadrine Spansules®). A generic form of dextroamphetamine is available for the tablets. The tablets generally last from three to four hours and must be given two or three times a day. The manufacturer of the long-acting form of the medicine states that the dose should be once a day; unfortunately, it appears to last less than eight hours and some patients require additional doses. In some children it is less effective than an equal amount of Dexedrine tablets. Desoxyn is available as a 5-milligram tablet. Adderall is available as 5-, 10-, 20-, and 30-milligram tablets. It is currently given as two doses a day. More experience will be needed to determine if, like Dexedrine and Desoxyn, three doses a day will be required for some children. Ritalin is available as 5-, 10-, and 20-

milligram tablets whose effects are somewhat shorter, perhaps lasting three hours or less. For this reason it is sometimes given twice a day and more usually must be given three times a day (morning, noon, and perhaps early afternoon) and sometimes even four times a day. A long-acting form of methylphenidate, Ritalin-SR, is available. The manufacturers had hoped that it would remain active for as long as eight hours and that it would have to be given only once or twice a day. Unfortunately, it seems to last no more than four hours and is less effective than the 20 milligrams. Another disadvantage is that it is available only in a 20–milligram form, which makes the fine-tuning of dosage impossible when it is used alone. The advantage of the long-acting forms of medication is that the child receives medication only once a day, in the morning; in contrast, the tablets usually have to be given two to four times a day. For the reasons mentioned above, however, using the current long-acting forms of medication is not always possible. Fortunately, formulations of Ritalin, which may last twelve hours, have been developed and should be available in the near future.

If the child is taking a medication whose effects last less than three to four hours, and he does not come home from school for lunch, the medication must be administered around noon at school and at about three or four o'clock in the afternoon. School nurses will administer the medication with a physician's note, although many children do not want to visit the nurse, because they are afraid that other children will identify them as being different. It is easy to see that, under these circumstances, a child may become negativistic about taking medication at all. If the child objects to taking medication at school, one may have to switch to one of the longer acting drugs such, as Dexedrine Spansules or the long-acting formulations of Ritalin that are being developed.

It is important for parents to realize that the effects of stimulant drugs last for only a brief period of time. For the amphetamines and methylphenidate there is no carryover from one day to the next. When the medication is effective, the parents will find that if it is discontinued for a day, the child's temperamental problems promptly reappear. Thus, the child's ADHD may be present in the morning until he receives his medication. If part of his problem is dawdling about getting dressed, eating breakfast, and going to school, it may be useful or necessary to give him the medication as soon as he awakens. Similarly, the effect of the medicine will wear off as the day goes on. If the medicine wears off at three or four o'clock and a parent's main contacts with the child are only after the child comes home from school, the parent may get the impression that the medicine is not helping. To check up on this, the parent should carefully observe the child's behavior on the weekend, at times when the medicine is most active—that is, mornings and early afternoons. This will also allow the parent to observe carefully how long each dose lasts and help the doctor to determine the best spacing of doses. Since the medicines are generally given in doses that permit the effects to wear off in the later afternoon or early evening, parents may anticipate more difficulty with the child at that time. If the child has to do homework after school or if parents are planning to take the child out in the evening or, say, to attend a large family gathering, it is often helpful to give a small additional dose later in the afternoon. As a rule this is not done routinely because these drugs tend to keep children awake.

After beginning with the smallest dose of medication that has been found useful with ADHD children, the physician will then usually follow the principle of increasing the medication until either the child's behavioral problems improve to what seems to be the greatest possible extent or the side effects of the increased dosages cause a problem in themselves. To determine how much benefit the child is receiving, the physician will want to know what is happening at home and at school. The schoolteacher is in an excellent position to determine the effects of medicine because he or she sees the child in circumstances in which he is apt to have the most difficulty. Furthermore, the teacher can compare his behavior with that of many other children of his age and intellectual ability. It is an excellent idea for the parent to stay in regular contact with the teacher, especially whenever the medication is being adjusted or changed. The parent should tell the teacher that the child is receiving treatment and should ask for a report on any changes the teacher may notice in the child's classroom behavior. Practically, it is useful not to make a big issue about this kind of information. Most people who expect to find changes tend to see them even if they are not present, so the parent should merely request information and not suggest that the teacher should expect to see the child improve. Another reason for not suggesting that the child may improve is that many teachers, trying to spare parents' feelings, will fail to report any difficulty the child may be having in school. If the child improves somewhat, and is now only a minor problem rather than a major problem, the teacher may inform the parent that things are going "pretty well." What the parent wants to know is if there are *any* problems, what kind they are, and how bad they are.

When the medicine is given will depend on the sorts of problems the ADHD child has. If the problems occur primarily in school, many physicians will prescribe the medicine only during the school week and not on weekends, holidays, and vacations. If there are problems both at school and at home, the physician will recommend that the medication be given every day. After the medicine has been taken for some time some physicians like to employ medication-free periods. This is done for two reasons. The first is to give the child a rest from medicine. Although there is no evidence that these medications are harmful, most physicians would prefer to give as little as possible of any medicine. A second reason for rest periods is to see if the child has outgrown his need for the medication. Sometimes, if ADHD symptoms diminish as the child grows older, he may only need the medication during stressful periods. That means that the medication can be stopped during school vacations. As the child becomes still older, the physician may want the child to begin school in the fall without medication and see how he does through the first few weeks. During this time the parents should, of course, stay in close touch with the school to see if problems are developing. If no problems emerge, that will provide considerable evidence that the ADHD child is outgrowing his problems. As previously emphasized, parents should always bear in mind that hyperactivity and restlessness themselves may disappear, whereas other problems, such as poor concentration and underachievement, may persist. The parents should therefore request detailed information from the teacher. Information that the child is not restless is not sufficient. How he is adjusting with his classmates, how he is concentrating on his tasks, and how much work he is able to do and how well must all be examined closely.

The purpose of giving medication is more than simply to control the child's behavior and allow him to adjust to an environment he does not like and in which he does poorly: school. Effective medication often affords the child self-control. In a sense he will have more, not less, freedom, and will suffer less from symptoms such as moodiness and anger. By being less bossy, more obedient (but not becoming a robot!), cooler tempered, and a better student, he will be better liked by teachers, parents, siblings, and peers. He will feel better about himself and about his life. More than his school performance improves. His life improves.

A final point. Unlike adults, children generally do *not* become tolerant of the effects of these medications, although it is common to see a small amount of tolerance develop during the first few weeks of treatment. In those instances one finds that a dosage of medication that for a month or so provided relief of symptoms gradually fails to control those symptoms. The physician will then usually increase the medication and find no further development of tolerance. Usually, if a child stays on the medication for several years, he may require an increased dose of medication as he becomes older and larger. In a few instances children do become tolerant to one of the stimulant drugs. In such circumstances most physicians then switch to another drug. Occasionally, it is necessary to alternate drugs in this manner. If the development of a drug tolerance continues to present a problem, the physician will often then switch to still another of the major categories of medications used.

Because the amphetamines and Ritalin can be abused by adults, their prescription is carefully monitored. They cannot be called into the pharmacist—he must receive a written prescription, only one month's supply may be prescribed at a time, and, as a result, a new prescription must be written each month. Cylert is much less abusable by adults and prescription restrictions are fewer. However, Cylert's potential severe toxicity presents a strong reason for not using it except in exceptional circumstances.

Side Effects

When given to children, the stimulant drugs—except Cylert— are unusually safe medications. [As mentioned earlier, there have been at least thirteen cases of acute liver failure and eleven deaths in patients taking Cylert. Blood tests of liver function cannot predict when this may occur. Such catastrophic side effects have not been reported with the amphetamines or Ritalin. Considering that the amphetamines and Ritalin have been given to many, many more patients than Cylert, the risks of the latter must be considered even greater.] Because the stimulants have opposite effects in children and non-ADHD adults (as noted, adults are made high and excited; children are not and often are made calm), the effect of these medications is sometimes called paradoxical. This is true only in some respects and not in others. In both children and adults the stimulant drugs decrease appetite and tend to interfere with sleep. Usually, but not always, the child's decreased appetite continues as long as medication is active and may be accompanied by some degree of weight loss. Although this weight loss may produce some concern in the parents, it never occurs to a medically serious degree. (Children's appetites generally return in the evening after the medication wears off. Accordingly, they should be allowed to eat after dinner and as much as they like. Appetite will also be normal, of course, at breakfast, before the medication has had time to act.) The drug's tendency to keep some children awake can usually be controlled by careful administration. Medication keeps children awake only while it is still in the bloodstream (that is, three to six hours after the last dose of pills and up to eighteen to twenty-four hours for the long-acting capsules). This is the reason for *not* giving these medications late in the day. If sleeplessness continues to be a problem, it can generally be handled by *not* using the long-acting form of the medicine and by being careful not to give the last pill too late in the day. When the medication is adjusted this way, sleeplessness will not be a problem. However, behavior problems may appear later in the day as the medication wears off. Insomnia can generally be avoided by having the last dose administered so as to wear off (in three or four hours) by the child's bedtime. If insomnia remains a problem and the child has difficulty with behavioral control at bedtime, the physician may recommend that the last dose be given earlier in the day. If insomnia constitutes a substantial problem, the physician may sometimes suggest the use of other drugs at bedtime. Both Mellaril (thioridazine) and Catapres (clonidine) are employed at bedtime. Mellaril is a "major tranquilizer." Unlike drugs like Valium, it is not abusable and patients do not become dependent on it. *Large* doses for *long* periods of time *may* produce neurological symptoms in some patients. These are very uncommon with lower doses, but patients receiving this medication should be followed regularly. These drugs chemically block the arousing effects of stimulants and thus allow the child to fall asleep. There are possible safety concerns with both drugs and their use should be discussed with the physician. Cylert has different side effects. In addition to possible (and uncommon) toxicity to the liver, it sometimes produces irritability and depression.

STIMULANT MEDICATIONS AND GROWTH

Several years ago a report was published stating that stimulant medications decreased the rate of growth—both of height and weight—in ADHD children. Since that report appeared, a number of other studies on the same subject have been published. It does appear that growth rate is slowed for a period of one or two years. After that, growth rate appears to approach normal. The whole issue is complicated because ADHD children may have growth patterns that are different from those of other children and the usual tables of growth may not apply to ADHD children. Doctors who have treated ADHD children with stimulants from childhood through adolescence have not observed any long-term effects of stimulant medication on height. When slowing of growth velocity occurs, this trend can be changed by the use of lower doses of medication and summer vacations from medicine. Research is being conducted to determine the exact effects of stimulant medication on growth.

There is no doubt that many ADHD children do lose weight on stimulant medication. Although this is sometimes upsetting to parents, there is no information suggesting that it is harmful, and weight usually returns to normal when the medication is stopped. I should reemphasize that the effects that have been reported are small and that most physicians treating ADHD children regard the psychological benefits as outweighing *possible* effects on the rate of growth. At a practical level, what the physician must do is follow the child's height, weight, and changes in adjustment and base the use of stimulant medication not only on its effect on growth but on its effects on the child's psychological well-being.

NONSTIMULANT DRUGS

Other medications sometimes used in the treatment of ADHD include those belonging to the groups called antidepressants, antihypertensives, and vitamins.

Antidepressants

First used in the treatment of ADHD children in the 1960s, the cyclic antidepressants include Elavil or Endep (amitriptyline), Tofranil (imipramine), and Norpramin (desipramine). They were formerly widely prescribed for the treatment of serious depression in adults, but for this treatment have been largely replaced by such drugs as Prozac, Zoloft, Paxil, Luvox, and Celexa—because they may be more effective and have fewer side effects. If the cyclic antidepressants are given to an adult who is not depressed or a child who does not have ADHD, they have little effect. They certainly do not produce a "high" nor are they habit forming. In fact, a normal adult or non-ADHD child would find the effects of these medications unpleasant and would not want to continue them.

During the 1980s, Wellbutrin (bupropion), an antidepressant with a different chemical structure from the cyclic antidepressants, received some testing among ADHD children but the drug company stopped the experiments and the drug has not been approved for use in children. Bupropion has also been used experimentally for the treatment of ADHD in adults, but until recently only in a few patients and not continuously. Larger experiments with adults have been performed and their results are awaited. Its effectiveness still remains to be determined.

There are three reasons why antidepressants are not widely used in children. The principal reason is that there have been a number of deaths in medically healthy ADHD children who were receiving one particular antidepressant, Norpramin (desipramine). The cyclic antidepressants can prolong the conduction of electrical activity in the heart; if this conduction becomes too slow, serious effects on the heart can occur. A second reason they are not widely used is that they appear to be less effective than the stimulant medications. Fewer children respond, although there is an occasional child who fails to respond to stimulants who does respond to these drugs. Generally in the children who respond, fewer ADHD symptoms appear to improve. Even in those children for whom they work at first, tolerance to the medication often develops; the medication stops working, and increasing the dose does not restore its therapeutic effects. (The tricyclic antidepressants may, however, be useful in the treatment of children who have both ADHD and another psychiatric illness.) The third reason they are not widely used is that, although they appear safe in depressed adults who may take them for years, it is not yet known what long-term effects they would have if used in the treatment of ADHD children over a period of years.

There are two major differences between their effects on depression in adults and on ADHD in children. First, rather than taking two to four weeks to work, in children the medications produce an effect in days. Second, by the time those antidepressants are having their maximal effect in adults (six to eight weeks), the ADHD children often have become tolerant to them. When this happens, increasing the dose worsens rather than betters the children's symptoms. It is the general opinion of child psychiatrists that in ADHD children who do not also have a biological depression, these drugs are of less value than the stimulants.

Dosage

The useful dose varies greatly and the physician will probably regulate it by obtaining blood tests to measure its level in the blood. Most children who take cyclic antidepressants require between 50 and 200 milligrams of them a day. Because susceptibility to the medicines varies widely from child to child, the physician will generally begin with a low dose and gradually increase it over a period of several weeks, until either the child's symptoms improve or the side effects of the medicine become unpleasant. In some instances the usefulness of the medicine is immediately apparent; in others, the parent must be prepared to wait several weeks before it can be determined whether the medicine is helpful.

Some antidepressants sometimes produce some sleepiness the first few weeks they are administered. The sleepiness generally goes away with the passage of time. Generally, the physician will have to wait until the child has developed a tolerance to the sleepiness before increasing the dose of the medication.

Side effects

The most important side effect of antidepressants is their effect on electrical conduction in the heart, as discussed earlier. To guard against this, electrocardiograms are taken before tricyclic antidepressants are begun and periodically thereafter. It is not known to what extent this monitoring can decrease the risks of their administration. In addition to sleepiness, antidepressants sometimes produce other unpleasant nondangerous side effects, such as irritability, dry mouth, lowered blood pressure when standing, constipation, and mild dizziness. These side effects usually diminish after a while or can be controlled by slightly lowering the dose. Antidepressants rarely produce allergy, but as a precautionary measure periodic blood tests may be performed.

Antihypertensives

Catapres (clonidine) is a drug developed for the treatment of hypertension (elevated blood pressure) that has been used in treating aggressive ADHD children and as a nighttime sedative in children who are receiving stimulants and in whom the stimulants produce insomnia. It is not abusable and appears to be of most use (but how much is uncertain) in very hyperactive or behaviorally disruptive children. It is ordinarily begun at a low dose (0.05 milligrams at bedtime) and increased as tolerated every third day. One formulation is available as a skin patch that releases doses over a period of a week. It is reported to require two weeks or so for its therapeutic action to begin. There have been a few reports of deaths that may have been caused by the combination of Ritalin and Catapres. Even though these deaths may have been coincidental, and not due to the drug combination, many child psychiatrists are reluctant to use the combination.

A relatively new drug, Tenex (guanfacine), which has an action similar to that of Catapres, has been reported to be useful in some ADHD children. Since it may lower blood pressure less and be less sedative, it may be more desirable. Its effectiveness remains to be determined.

Vitamins

In the past, a few physicians have suggested the use of very large doses of vitamins in the treatment of children and adults with psychiatric difficulties, describing megavitamin therapy as a safe and effective treatment for several kinds of behavioral disorders. At present all one can say is that these claims are unsubstantiated. Nevertheless, the parent might believe that a trial use of large doses of vitamins would at least be natural and therefore safe. The difficulty is that although the vitamins are natural, doses of ten to a thousand times the normal daily requirement are not natural and may not be safe. Salt and water are natural, but someone who drinks many times the normal requirement of water a day might well die of water intoxication. Although further information may show megavitamin therapy to be effective and safe, there is now no evidence affirming that it is effective, and more evidence is needed to indicate that it is safe.

There are many other medications that sometimes prove effective when the above substances do not work. In some instances a physician may have to try several, and the parents may have to wait several months before finding out if there is a medication that will benefit the child. No medication used in the treatment of ADHD children is ideal—each has some disadvantages, usually minor. Researchers are constantly working to improve them, but in the meantime the available medications are usually effective (often dramatically so) and safe, and in the large majority of instances their advantages completely outweigh their disadvantages.

AIDS TO ADMINISTERING MEDICINE

Many parents do not realize it, but there are important psychological aspects to giving and taking medicine. This is usually overlooked because most medications are either for medical conditions or for obvious psychological ones. People take aspirin because of a headache, laxatives because of constipation, and tranquilizers because of anxiety. The how's and why's are straightforward. But in the administration of medicine to children for ADHD, several psychological principles play an important role. If treatment is to be maximally effective, these principles must be properly applied.

First, the child must have some understanding of why he is receiving medication. Second, he must be assured that taking medicine does not mean that his problems are terrible, such as being brain damaged or crazy. Third, it is useful to have him recognize and acknowledge problems in his own behavior *that he himself does not like,* so that he will not feel that medicine is being given to him simply so that other people can tolerate him more. If a child does not understand why he is receiving medication, if he does not feel that he has problems and that the medicine is helping him with these problems, he is likely to resist taking it, forget to take it, or discontinue it when he grows older but may still need it.

Usually an ADHD child will recognize and acknowledge certain features of his experience and behavior that he does not like or that get him into trouble. These may include such things as not being able to pay attention, having a hot temper, being "nervous" (restless), or being criticized by teachers or parents for forgetting things, not finishing work, or being out of the classroom seat all the time. He can honestly be told that the medicine will help him to complete his schoolwork, pay attention, hold his temper, be less nervous, remember things better, and to calm down. If he can accept the fact that the medicine is helping him, a large task has been accomplished. He will feel that something is being done for him rather than to him.

It is also important in giving medicine to children that they do not get the idea that because they have to take medicine they are somehow excused from assuming responsibility for their own behavior. ADHD, like any other illness, does not negate free will. It may limit or modify someone's behavioral options, but it does not eliminate all responsibility. Children *can and must feel* that they share a responsibility for their behavior. They should not attribute all their actions to powers beyond their control. They should not be allowed to play the kind of "game" that Eric Berne, in his book *Games People Play*, calls wooden leg. In this psychological game, the person says the equivalent of "What can you expect of me? I couldn't do more. I've got a wooden leg." Children should be prevented from adopting the same attitude with regard to their ADHD. They should not be allowed to imply: "I am a psychological cripple. I have ADHD. All my actions are beyond my own control." For this reason, parents (and teachers and brothers and sisters as well) should not explain the ADHD child's behavior on the basis of whether or not he's taken his medication. Parents should not say to him: "You're acting up. When did you have your medicine?" Putting things this way leads the child to believe that he has no control of himself, and it may place him in the position of having his "badness" explained by the absence of medicine and his "goodness" explained by its presence. If so, he can take no credit for controlling himself, and when he has not behaved in an appropriate way, he frequently can excuse himself because he hasn't taken his medication. If in talking to the ADHD child, his parents, teachers, or brothers and sisters often associate his behavior with his medication schedule, he soon will learn how to play the game of "medicine wooden leg": "What can you expect of me? I have ADHD and my medicine wore off."

The importance of communicating to children their responsibility for their own behavior will become clearer in the section of this chapter entitled "Psychological Management."

DIETARY TREATMENT

■

As I mentioned in Chapter 3, some physicians have suggested that ADHD may be due to bodily reactions to normal food constituents. One possibility is that some children may be allergic to certain foods and the allergy may produce behavioral problems. A second, and different, claim was made by a California physician, Dr. Ben Feingold (*Why Your Child Is Hyperactive*, Random House, 1975), who believes that many children develop ADHD as a reaction to artificial colorings, flavorings, some preservatives (which may be present in processed foods), and salicylates (a chemical related to aspirin) that are found naturally in some fruits and vegetables. A diet that eliminates these chemicals is called a food-additive-free or Feingold diet. The idea that food additives might cause ADHD is particularly appealing to those people who believe that food additives are "unnatural" (and therefore probably harmful), and that treatment with a special, healthful diet seems preferable to treatment with drugs. When children are put on these special diets without any attempt to disguise the treatment, some children do seem to show significant change in behavior. This is probably due to the change in the family's attitude about that child (which usually means more time spent with that child) and hopeful expectations in the minds of the child and his family. However, all the carefully conducted, controlled studies—in which the family does not know whether or not the child is on the additive-free diet—have shown that one type of additive (the artificial food colorings) does not produce significant hyperactivity (though it may produce some minor changes in attention in some children). Because there is still some room to hope that the food-additive-free diet may help *some* children, there would be no harm in families trying this special diet, as long as they pay attention to good nutrition and remain particularly alert to the need for vitamin C. (The Feingold diet limits the intake of several popular vitamin-C-containing fruits.) So far, however, I remain pessimistic about any relationship between food additives and ADHD.

The subject of food allergies remains controversial. Some physicians believe that food allergies are frequently the cause of behavioral problems, while many others either doubt the existence of food allergies or think they occur infrequently and usually only in infants and toddlers. Doctors argue about this issue because there are no laboratory tests that can diagnose whether a food allergy exists. Therefore, the diagnosis must be made on the basis of clinical judgment—which means there is room for disagreement. Most physicians agree that the only certain way to diagnose food allergies is through an elimination diet. This usually involves removing all but the most basic, simple foods from the child's diet and then gradually, one at a time, adding foods back and observing the child's reaction. This is a tedious and time-consuming process that requires much patience on the part of both child and parent. For that reason, there has to be fairly good evidence that allergy may be a problem before most physicians are willing to try the elimination diet. It is my impression, as mentioned in Chapter 3, that the symptoms of food allergy are really different from the symptoms of true ADHD. An occasional ADHD child *may* show improvement if he is found to be allergic to certain foods and is placed on a diet that does not contain them. If parents think that food allergies may be causing problems for their child, it is probably a good idea for them to seek a physician's help in identifying possible allergies and then placing the child on a special diet that does not include the targeted foods. Although some pediatricians will investigate the child's possible food allergies, many would prefer that the child be seen by a pediatric allergist. It is important for parents to realize, however, that at present there is little evidence that food allergies play any substantial role in the behavior problems associated with hyperactivity.

COFFEE

A few years ago someone proposed that ADHD might be less common in South American countries—which may or may not be true—because children there drank coffee. Because coffee contains caffeine, a recognized stimulant of the brain, and because stimulants seem to help ADHD, it was inferred that caffeine might be useful in treating ADHD. A few studies have been conducted and they seem to indicate that caffeine, by itself, is *not* useful in treating ADHD. When caffeine is combined with stimulant drug treatment, the overall response is better than with stimulant drugs alone, but the same good response can be obtained simply by increasing the amount of the stimulant drug. Because caffeine is less effective than the stimulant medication and has a variety of side effects that are considered undesirable, coffee does not have a useful place in the treatment of the ADHD child.

PSYCHOLOGICAL MANAGEMENT

■

Most ADHD children can benefit from medication. All of them can benefit from understanding and consistent parenting and care. ADHD children have special problems, but like all other children they may have "unspecial" ones as well. Difficulties, misunderstandings, friction between parent and child will cause trouble for any child, but they may cause more trouble for the ADHD child. This book focuses on the particular psychological problems the ADHD child is likely to develop because of his difficulties in the areas of attention, impulsivity, and hyperactivity.

UNDERSTANDING THE PROBLEM

The first part of this book has been devoted to a description of the typical problems of the ADHD child and why he has these problems. It is very difficult to understand that a child who is attention-demanding, contrary, and short tempered may be having a physical problem. Intuitively, one believes that he is having a psychological problem. As I have tried to make clear, he does have psychological problems but they are physically caused.

If this is so, how should a parent handle the problems? It seems that, if a problem is psychological, the child is responsible for his behavior. If he is good he should be praised, and if he is bad he should be punished. Similarly, if the problem is physical, the child is not responsible for his behavior. If that is so, he should not be rewarded for being good or punished for being bad. Neither of the above beliefs is true. Temperament may influence behavior, but it is not the only factor that determines behavior. Temperament may make it easier or harder for a child to control himself. It may make it easier for him to learn to respond to discipline. But how the parents feel about the child and how they treat him can have appreciable effects.

During the past few years psychiatrists and psychologists have found that patients whose severe psychological problems are physically caused can benefit markedly from psychological treatment. Down's Syndrome, a severe form of retardation, is physically caused, but certain techniques of training can teach children with this disorder more effectively. Psychosis, severe psychological disturbances in adults, may produce childlike, withdrawn, or destructive behavior. These patients, whose symptoms are worse than those of any ADHD child, can in many cases be helped by certain techniques. These techniques are based on three principles: (1) making the patients responsible for their behavior; (2) rewarding them for good behavior; (3) punishing them (in a special way) for bad behavior.

Similarly, the ADHD child does better when he is held accountable and made responsible for his behavior. He should not be allowed to say, either in so many words or indirectly, "I'm ADHD—I'm a mental cripple—I'm not responsible for what I do." He should be treated as responsible and, if necessary, be told something to this effect: "You do have problems that may sometimes make it hard for you to control yourself. But the same thing is true for everybody. Everyone does some things more easily than others and does other things with more difficulty. You can learn to [count to ten, hold your temper, not tease your sister] and I expect you to." As with all my suggestions, of course, parents should change the words to suit themselves and their children.

The child should not be held to be either irresponsible or blameworthy and should be treated as someone who has a greater tendency than average to do certain things. On the other hand, the parents should realize that for most ADHD children no method of child-rearing would eliminate certain tendencies. The child will tend to be more attention-seeking and forgetful, and will seem absentminded and willful. In most instances he is not doing these things to annoy. He would do them no matter how he had been raised. This distinction between symptoms that can be benefited by both rearing and medicine and those that can be alleviated only by medicine is important to remember. It will prevent parents from trying to use psychological methods to change things that cannot be changed (or at best changed very little) in this way. Although psychologically unchangeable symptoms vary from child to child, they usually include the following: short attention span, distractibility, moodiness, lack of stick-to-itiveness, school underachievement, and immaturity. They *may* include bed-wetting, soiling, and some antisocial behaviors such as stealing. Again, remember that although psychological techniques may not completely eliminate these problems in the child, they may help him. For example, the child may continue to have tantrums, but he can be taught what to do when he has them. This will be discussed later.

In summary, parents must remember three things. One, the child does have difficulties in doing and not doing certain things. Two, he will learn best how to compensate for his problems if he is treated as a responsible person who can gradually learn to control himself and his behavior. Three, the degree to which his problems can be helped by particular child-rearing techniques varies. It is much easier to teach him how to control his temper or how to take responsibility for his chores than to teach him to have a longer attention span or to be less distractible. Both medicine and discipline will help the first kind of problem (e.g., temper, and chores). The second kind of problem (e.g., short attention span) for the most part can be helped only by medicine.

BASIC PROCEDURES

The main problem of the ADHD child at home involves discipline. In discussing the basic procedures that will help the child to function effectively in his home environment, I will first indicate how the parents can establish constructive rules for the child. The second section will describe the rewards and punishments most likely to ensure that the child will adhere to these rules.

Establishing Rules

Considerable evidence exists that certain ways of handling ADHD children are more effective than others. It has been found that a firm, consistent, explicit, predictable home environment is the best. Let me elaborate the special meaning that these terms have with respect to disciplining the ADHD child. *Firm* means that rules or expectations for the child always have the same consequences. If he breaks a particular rule, he is always punished and always in the same way. If he does what he is asked, he always obtains acknowledgment or praise. *Consistent* means that the rules themselves do not change from day to day. If he is supposed to clean up his room before going out to play, he is never allowed to leave his room until it has been cleaned up. *Explicit* means clearly defined and clearly understood by all parties. For example, cleaned up could mean that clothes have been hung in the closet, or that the bed has been made, or that toys have been returned to a shelf, or that the room has been vacuumed and dusted, or any combination of these. For the cleaning-up rule, the definition of cleaning up must be explicit enough so that the child and the parents understand the rule the same way. *Predictable* means that the laws are made before, not after, the crime.

Obviously, all parental expectations for the child cannot be stated beforehand. Parents never consider telling the toddler not to put nail polish on the rug and rarely think of telling him not to put a toy car in his ear. Some things can be dealt with only after they happen. In general, however, for most daily activities, rules can and should be made and then enforced. The child must wash himself, brush his teeth, do his around-the-house chores and homework every day; rules concerning these routine functions should be established. Punishment should follow any violation of the rules, but should not be employed if the rules have not been agreed on beforehand. Analogous consistent and predictable rules for adults exist in the speed limits for driving. It is easier to abide by a specific speed limit, say 55 mph, than adhere to the vague limit, "reasonable and proper," that was formerly designated in some Western states. In the case of the vague speed limit one does not know how fast one can go if it is twilight and a light rain is falling. Someone who is fearful may drive 35 mph. Someone who is more adventurous and drives at 40 mph may rightly be upset when she gets a ticket.

The above suggestions may impress parents as harsh and possibly cruel. They may also seem to contradict various benign permissive doctrines that advocate allowing children to "do their own thing," and allow opportunities for parents and children to talk things over. Let me correct some common misconceptions. First, firmness is not the same as harshness. Harshness is excessively severe or brutal rule enforcement. It is harsh to imprison someone for life for driving too fast. It is firm to fine him every time he does so. Second, children need structure. They need established rules, expectations, and values by which to live. Such structure does not mean the absence of freedom.

All people living in society have to follow certain rules and expectations if that society is to function effectively. Adults must not steal, drive when drunk, or embezzle. They must not urinate in public. Behaving in accordance with such rules also benefits the individual. First, and obviously, it keeps him out of trouble. But it also helps some individuals directly. Someone who has only poorly learned to control his impulses must consume a large part of his energy in simply controlling himself. The reformed alcoholic or drug addict must expend a great deal of effort in preventing himself from backsliding. The person who has learned to control himself readily has energies that he can utilize profitably elsewhere.

Note that this is not contrary to self-expression or creativity. The person who is brilliant but cannot focus his energies will not be productive (consider the old saw that genius is 1 percent inspiration and 99 percent perspiration). Firm, consistent rules for behavior have nothing at all to do with the child's self-expression or with understanding between parent and child. I have been talking about rules for behavior, not rules for thoughts and feelings. Thoughts and feelings are very different from behavior. They cannot be regulated and the parent should not attempt to regulate them. As discussed later, parents should help their children acknowledge and express their feelings. But both the parent and the child should always discriminate between feelings and behavior. For example, the parents of an ADHD child should allow him to express his jealous feelings toward his newborn sister, but he should not be allowed to hit her. Feeling jealous and hitting because of jealousy should be recognized as being as different as night and day.

Finally, the setting of firm rules need not interfere with helpful discussions between the parents and the child. As the child becomes older such discussions certainly should be a part of family life, but even when he is younger they may be helpful. The child may, for example, suggest ways of getting his tasks done in a way that he likes better and that does not compromise the family. This is perfectly acceptable and in fact should be encouraged. But talking things over should not prevent rules from being formulated. It may influence how they are decided on and it may modify their exact terms, but it should not interfere with their being established explicitly and consistently.

What evidence is there that the kind of structure discussed here is useful? Very interesting information comes from a study done in the mid-1930s with severely "hyperactive" children. The behavior of these children was so uncontrollable at home that they had to be placed in a hospital for children with serious behavior problems. The physicians had no previous experience with such children and tried various techniques to see which would be most effective. They began by assuming that the problems of the children were the result of excessive emotional stress and strain, and they treated them with a great deal of tolerance. This technique produced a brief period of improvement, which was soon followed by a recurrence of the same behavioral problems. Next, since the children had never received psychotherapy, they were treated in individual psychotherapy. This approach, too, proved unsuccessful. Finally, the doctors decided to create an environment that was "constructive," "restrictive," and "tolerant." The rules were not lax, and definite compliance to them was expected of the children. Children were isolated but not criticized for impulsive behavior (I will discuss this isolation later), and after they had calmed down they were helped to express themselves. The last technique clearly produced the greatest benefit, and many children could be discharged from the hospital to their homes. Unfortunately, those children who returned to homes in which parents could not be firm often again became disturbed and had to return to the hospital. It is important to emphasize that not all children benefited by this (or any other) technique, but it was the technique that worked best.

This and similar studies give us evidence that environments structured in such ways can help ADHD children. There is also reason to believe that they are most effective if begun early in life and are relatively ineffective (perhaps useless) if initiated later in childhood. The techniques to be discussed may help the preschool or young school-aged child a great deal. They may be totally ineffective with an ADHD child who is approaching adolescence.

What the specific rules should be in a particular family depend on parental preference and the age of the child. Parents could theoretically make any rules and teach young children to abide by them. (Different cultures have vastly different rules and standards for child behavior, and each culture succeeds in making a "standard product," a child well adapted to living in that culture.) As the child grows older, the parents' latitude in setting these rules decreases. The young child is for the most part only aware of how his own family does things. The older child is very much aware of how other children and their families do things, and will tend to rebel if his parents' standards appear different. A mother may keep her two-year-old boy in long curls and he will not protest. But it would be foolish of her to try to give her fourteen year old a prep-school-style haircut if his friends look like the latest rock idol. The earlier that rules and values are taught to a child the more likely he will be to maintain them later, even in the face of different standards outside the family.

The techniques to be discussed work best on younger children, say, up to the age of ten or eleven. These methods, which require that the child is still dependent on and controlled by his parents, are not for teenagers—they need a different psychological approach.

With younger children, the first task for parents is to decide, concretely and specifically, what behaviors require limitations or change. It is important to be concrete and specific so that the rules can be stated clearly and explicitly. Let me give some examples of vague, meaningless rules and how they can be clarified.

A. "He should clean his room." As I have indicated, this rule is highly ambiguous. If by "cleaning the room" the parent means put everything away and the child understands make your bed, he can feel wronged if he makes his bed, leaves, and is criticized. Furthermore, there is room for endless debate. The child cleaned the room by his standards but did not clean it by his mother's. We will return to this particular topic later in the subsection entitled "Chores."

B. "He should have better table manners." This might mean: he should eat with his fork instead of his fingers; he should put a napkin on his lap; he should say "please"; he should not use a boardinghouse reach.

C. "He should treat his little sister better." This could mean: he should not hit her; he should allow her to play with his toys; he should not retaliate if she hits him.

D. "He should be neater." This might mean: he should tie his shoelaces; button his shirt; wash his face; brush his teeth.

Not only does the child not know what his parents mean if they are not specific—and he can and will argue with them in the best legalistic fashion about what they might have meant—but also parents will have a much harder time determining whether progress has really taken place.

The second task of parents is to establish a hierarchy of importance for the rules. They must decide what is essential, what is important, what would be nice, and what is trivial. The parents must decide what are five-star rules and which are one-star ones. They must fit the punishment to the crime; they must distinguish between felonies and misdemeanors. They must not, so to speak, punish illegal parking with life imprisonment and punish murder with a warning. For example, parents have been known to use a talk as punishment for the setting of a serious fire and a severe spanking as punishment for poor homework. The usefulness of establishing five- and one-star rules is that it helps parents concentrate on the more important areas first and gives the child some breathing room. After the most essential problems have been brought under control, the parents can move to the next category.

Another task for the parents is to predecide that both mother and father will abide by the prescribed course of action. This policy is not always easy to carry out. Frequently, each parent has devised his or her own (usually not too successful) technique for dealing with the child, and unfortunately each often believes that that technique is right and the child's problems are the result of the other's mismanagement. If such a family atmosphere exists, it conflicts with the consistent united front that is an absolute requirement for helping the ADHD child learn to control his behavior. It is not necessary for the parents to agree completely with each other—they simply must act in common. If parents are incapable of resolving their differences and agreeing on rules and standards for their ADHD child's behavior, they may benefit from psychological assistance. A psychiatrist, social worker, or psychologist may enable them to thrash out these differences and determine the set of rules, and the relative importance of the various rules, necessary for their ADHD child.

Rewards and Punishments

In addition to establishing sound rules to help the child, parents must predecide a plan of rewards and punishments. These rewards and punishments should be seen as such by the child and not only by the parents. The words reward and punishment have an unfortunate meaning to some people. Reward seems to suggest bribery and punishment to suggest brutality. All that is meant by reward is something the child likes, particularly attention, praise, or a small special privilege. Certain privileges, toys, and so forth can be useful under special conditions, which will be discussed later.

Similarly, punishment simply means something the child does not like. It does not mean beating, emotional neglect, or denial of privileges for a long time. Generally, with younger children, a most effective and nonhurtful punishment is sending the child to his room until he stops behaving in an undesirable way (e.g., having a tantrum) or finishes a required task (e.g., getting dressed). It is more effective to say, "Go to your room, please, and come back to breakfast when your shoes are tied and your face is washed," than it is to yell at the child or beat him.

There are two more important principles of reward and punishment. First, to be most useful, a reward or punishment should be immediate. Any delay decreases effectiveness. When a child does what you want him to, praise him on the spot. If he does what he has been told not to do, punish him at once. Do not offer distant presents ("any toy you want two weeks from now") or threaten punishment ("Daddy will spank you when he gets home"). Second, the one-time rule should be adopted. The parents should learn the habit of saying do or don't only *once* before rewarding or punishing. If they do not apply this rule, if they give first, second, third, and tenth warnings before acting, their children will learn to commit ten violations before worrying. In the meantime the parents will have developed sore throats and built up a good deal of angry steam. In some cases, the child may have been anxiously pushing his parent to take a stand. Surprisingly, most children are relieved when the parent finally acts. A good deal of friction can be avoided by the use of this one-time rule.

In the past forty years, psychologists have learned a great deal about reward and punishment from animal experimentation. Researchers have discovered extremely simple and effective techniques that can be used to teach animals, such as pigeons and rats, to perform very complicated tasks. For example, it is fairly easy to teach a rat to push a bar for food when a certain colored light is on. Using these techniques, one can teach a rat to push a bar very slowly for food under one set of conditions and very rapidly under another set.

Since then, psychologists have found that such techniques, called "operant conditioning," or behavioral modification, are sometimes helpful in teaching and controlling the behavior of human beings whose psychological difficulties are so great that previously they seemed unreachable by any known technique—for example, profoundly retarded children and adults, children of normal intelligence who are unable to talk, and seriously disturbed adult psychiatric patients. In more recent years a number of psychologists have tried applying these "operant" techniques to children with behavioral problems. The operant techniques—or operant conditioning—are no more than refined sets of rewards and punishments, and the work of the psychologists can be translated into recommendations that can be very helpful to parents of ADHD children.

The exact rules and laws of operant conditioning as they are used in the laboratory are somewhat complicated, but the basic principle that parents can use is exceedingly simple. It is that *acts are influenced by their consequences*. That is, what happens after an animal or child does something greatly influences, either positively or negatively, the likelihood of his doing the same thing again. For the parents, this means that how they act when their child does or says something will either increase or decrease the probability that the child will behave that way again.

This principle is most easy to illustrate in the use of operant conditioning with animals. In a typical experiment a hungry rat is placed in a simple cage with a bar in it. In the course of his explorations the rat eventually leans on the bar. When he does so a pellet of food is released automatically into the feeding dish. If one observes the rat through a one-way screen one sees that the rat may not return to the bar for a while. Eventually, perhaps by accident, he will depress the bar again, and again will be rewarded by food. As one continues to watch the rat, one finds that he eventually seems to get the idea. After a day or two of training in such a cage the hungry rat will immediately go to the bar and press it. Notice that I use the phrase *gets the idea*. Obviously there is no information about the consciousness of rats, and the phrase may be somewhat misleading, but in humans such behavior can be learned without awareness: some experiments seem to indicate that subjects may learn to change some kinds of behavior with no awareness whatsoever of the sequence that produces the change. That is, people may develop habits that produce certain consequences for them without being aware of any relationship between the habits, the acts based on those habits, and the consequences of those acts.

To illustrate the principle in animal experimentation again, I will describe a typical demonstration in an elementary psychology course. A hungry pigeon is placed in a cage. Standing outside the cage and observing the pigeon through a one-way screen is the experimenter. In his hand he holds a switch that he can use to cause a click to be made in the box and a kernel of corn delivered to the pigeon in a feeding dish. The experimenter may choose to make the pigeon perform any behavior pigeons are capable of. In one instance it was decided to make the pigeon rotate counterclockwise, spinning like a ballerina. In order to accomplish this, the experimenter waited until the pigeon in his normal wanderings had turned slightly to the left. After the pigeon had done so, the experimenter pressed the switch and the pigeon received a kernel of corn. In the next twenty or thirty seconds the pigeon again turned to the left, and the experimenter delivered another kernel of corn. In the following few minutes the pigeon began to rotate slowly toward his left. After he had done so for a while the experimenter again delivered a kernel of corn. During the next five or ten minutes the pigeon began to turn continuously in a circle. The experimenter would wait until the pigeon was turning rapidly and then, and only then, deliver the food. Thereafter, when the pigeon turned slowly he received no food and when he turned rapidly he received the food. At the end of the half-hour the class was astonished to see a pigeon rotating like a whirling dervish. This experiment illustrates the complex tasks that can be taught even to animals. More complex behavior can be taught to humans, and (as cannot be illustrated by animal experiments) such learning can apparently occur without the person's awareness of it as well as with his being conscious of it.

Before examining the question of what relevance these experiments have for people, let me digress for just a moment and define two, and only two, terms from operant conditioning therapy. The first term is operant, and the second is reinforcement. An operant is any voluntary act an animal or human being is capable of performing. It includes the rat's bar-pressing and the pigeon's circling. In fact, it includes most behaviors. In children it might even include talking, attention-getting, having tantrums, waking up in the middle of the night, lying, stealing, crying, fire-setting, writing poems, or philosophizing—in short, almost anything. Reinforcement is synonymous with the word reward. In the animal experiments discussed, reinforcement was food. Food is rewarding or reinforcing to a hungry animal.

What is reinforcing to children? That depends on their state. To the rat that has eaten his fill, food is no longer reinforcing and he will not depress a bar to obtain it. For a thirsty child, water can be reinforcing; for a hungry child, food can be reinforcing. However, most of the child's acts are influenced by parental behavior that is quite different from simple satisfaction of hunger or thirst. For an individual child, reinforcing behavior varies, *but certain parental acts and behaviors are reinforcing to almost all children.* The most important, as I have suggested, are parental affection and parental attention. Parental attention is probably the single most common reinforcer in a child's daily life. It is important not only because of the frequency with which it is focused on the child, but also because it is reinforcing no matter what elicits it. Some kinds of punishment, therefore, are more rewarding to a child than ignoring him. Expressing disapproval of a child's most recent misdeed is giving him attention. Thus, paradoxically, the likelihood that a child will repeat a misdeed may be increased when the parent discusses the misdeed with the child at too great a length.

What about more severe punishment? The reinforcers I have discussed are referred to by psychologists as positive reinforcers. What the layperson refers to as punishment, the psychologist calls negative reinforcement. Certain general principles have been learned about the effects and effectiveness of negative reinforcement.

To begin with, negative reinforcement *generally* reduces the likelihood of the repetition of the act that preceded it. Thus, as generations of parents have learned, with most children most of the time a "good spanking" was a pretty effective way of preventing a child from doing again what he just did that the parents didn't like. The rat that received a powerful electric shock after pressing the bar will refrain from doing so in the future or, at least, in the very near future. Psychologists have also learned some less obvious things about punishment. If it is very severe (e.g., a very painful electric shock, which is almost enough to paralyze the animal), the animal is likely *never* to repeat the act again, but punishments of this nature are also likely to be accompanied by side effects that change the animal in a number of undesirable ways. Animals that receive such powerful punishment are apt to become erratic and often show disturbed (neurotic) behavior in other areas. In experiments in which electric shocks have been used to teach dogs to avoid things, the dogs have become vicious, excited, withdrawn, or very fearful. In other words, punishment that is effective enough to prevent offensive behavior permanently may produce more disturbing behavior than what it prevented.

Thus, some punishment focuses attention on the child and therefore reinforces poor behavior, and if severe punishment is likely to produce bad side effects, the question arises as to whether any form of punishment can be reasonably effective. Although psychologists disagree, it seems that there are lesser degrees of punishment that can suppress behavior but only temporarily. That is, shocks that will not make the animal neurotic are not likely to be effective for very long. The relevance of this for children should be fairly obvious. Humane parents use only moderate punishment and, in ADHD children, who are often not particularly responsive to punishment, the effects of punishment should not be expected to be long lasting. And in fact they rarely are.

Positive reinforcement, on the other hand, may not be permanent either, but with certain modifications may be extremely long lasting. Its virtue is that once the child is started on the right track he is likely to receive reinforcement from people outside the family. The child who is taught to be reasonably polite, moderately obedient, and reasonably nonaggressive will be reinforced by favorable attention from others, by making friends and succeeding.

One other feature of positive reinforcement increases the possibility that it may have very long-lasting effects and it too can be illustrated by animal experimentation. When a rat is trained to push a bar, he receives food on every bar press. If one stops delivering a pellet each time the rat presses the bar, after a while the rat pushes less and less frequently and eventually stops. However, with a simple modification of the experiment, the rat can be made to work a much longer time for fewer pellets. Let us suppose we arrange the machine so that at first the rat receives a pellet only on every second bar push. Then after a while we arrange it so that he receives a pellet on every third, and every fourth, and so on. Now suppose we tinker around with the machinery (and this is very simple) so that the rat is playing a slot machine, that is, he receives a pellet, *on the average*, on every 20th or 50th or 100th bar press. Sometimes he receives three pellets in a row. Sometimes he may have to press the bar 200 times before receiving a pellet. After a rat has been exposed to this payoff system he is very resistant to losing his habit. Again the relevance of this to children should be obvious. One begins by reinforcing a child every time he performs a desired behavior. After a while one changes the payoff and gradually reinforces him less often for the same behavior. Like the rat in which reinforcement has been tapered off in the same way, the child is now likely to persist in this behavior even without a constant payoff.

Having criticized punishment (and not for humane grounds but for practical grounds), I must back down a little and point out that it does have some effectiveness and that it can be important in situations that are dangerous or life-threatening. The two year old rushing out into the street (to possible death) should be punished fairly severely and immediately. This will decrease the likelihood of his doing it again in the near future. One is more likely to keep him out of the street, however, if he is positively reinforced for doing things that prevent his going there (e.g., staying on the lawn or playing in the backyard). Punishment is a good temporary technique, but it is ineffective in the long run in most ADHD children. Even though punishment may be absolutely necessary (as for the two year old just mentioned), punishment should be as mild and as infrequently used as possible.

One point I've touched on but must emphasize is the question of when reinforcement should occur. One word will suffice: immediately. In the experiments with animals, the success of the technique depends on the animal's receiving the reinforcement the moment after the act—the operant—is performed. A delay of two seconds decreases its effectiveness a little, a delay of five seconds reduces it considerably, and a delay of a minute makes it useless. Children apparently can tolerate longer delays but the same principle applies to them. Positive reinforcement (or reward) and negative reinforcement (or punishment) are much more effective if they are received immediately. If a child does what the parent wants him to do, he should receive praise for that act immediately. If he does something that requires punishment, he should be punished immediately. It is ineffective and a waste of time to promise to reward a child in two weeks if he obtains good grades now or to delay necessary punishment until Daddy comes home. Such reinforcements *may* work at best temporarily (two weeks, or the rest of the day) but will have no long-lasting effect.

From this discussion the question emerges of how these techniques should be applied practically to children. They may be used informally and formally. Clearly, an important principle of their informal application is that children should be positively reinforced, immediately, when they do what their parents want. Once the child knows what his parents' desires are (e.g., putting his shoes away, eating with a fork, saying "please"), he should be reinforced by his parents in a specific way whenever he performs these acts. By specific I mean that the parents should comment on the desired behavior in believable and pertinent terms. If he is asked to put his shoes away and does so, the parent should not say, "You are a wonderful son." The parent should say, "I am very pleased that you are learning to take care of your things like a grown-up boy," or words to that effect. Children, like adults, recognize overgenerous praise as false. The child should know what he is receiving praise for.

Theoretically, the corresponding principle to be applied when children behave undesirably would require that the children are ignored, but how can the parent ignore undesirable behavior? If the child is acting like a clown, it is easy. If he is pummeling his three-year-old sister or destroying the house, ignoring him is dangerous or expensive. If he is engaging in harmless attention-seeking behavior, ignoring is easy. If he is engaged in behavior that is destructive or harmful, ignoring should be combined with the isolation-room technique.

The usefulness of the isolation room becomes apparent when one considers what ordinarily happens when a child misbehaves. For example, if the child punches his sister, the parent is apt to ask at least, "Why did you do that?" Thus, the child receives attention for misbehaving. In accordance with the principles discussed, attention is likely to increase the probability that the child will do the same thing again. In other words, the parents' normal discussion with the child is likely to result in greater future misbehavior. With the isolation-room technique, the child is informed beforehand that whenever he misbehaves he will be sent to his room. Then when he actually does misbehave he is simply told that he is going to his room and that he will be allowed to come out as soon as he regains control of himself. If he goes willingly, that is fine. If he has to be carried, that may not be fine but is effective. If he tries to leave his room, a screen-door latch should be placed on the outside of the door and locked.* When the child quiets down or—in the case of the older child—when he announces that he has quieted down

---

*Parents should *never* leave the house while the child is locked in the room because of the always present (even though remote) possibility of fire or similiar emergency.

and comes out himself, then, and only then, does the parent sit down with the child and discuss what was bothering him before. With this technique the child receives attention for being in control of himself, not for being out of control. After a child has had considerable experience with this procedure, he often learns to go to his room when he has become upset and come out when he is no longer upset. If the child has to be kept in the room, the parents should not let him out until he is able to be in control of himself—that is, until his tantrum has stopped or his anger outburst is under control. This technique has been used effectively with very disturbed hospitalized psychiatric patients as well as with ADHD children. It is an especially effective technique with young (under the age of nine or ten) ADHD children.

The second way in which reinforcement therapy can be applied, the more formal way, cannot be used with the youngest ADHD children, but is effective with children beyond, say, the age of six. With this method the parent and the child decide what tasks the parents would like the child to perform. These may be tasks that occur each day or once a week. They may, for example, include making his bed, putting his clothes in the hamper, or taking out the trash. A weekly chart is kept and the parent and the child predecide how many tokens—for example, poker chips—the child will receive for performing as agreed. Whenever the child does do the work, he promptly receives the predecided number of poker chips. The child is allowed to accumulate the credits he earns for desirable behavior and can exchange them later for objects or privileges he regards as desirable. In other words, he earns tokens and spends them for the movies, going out to play, watching TV, or, if the parents choose, even for money. In any event, the rate of exchange should also be decided on beforehand. This technique will be further described in the subsection entitled "Chores."

Contingency Contracting

Contingency contracting is a behavioral technique more suited for use with older children. The notion is very simple. Parents and children discuss what each desires from the other in very specific terms. In one example, a child's obligation might be cleaning up his room each morning, and the reward from the parent might be permission to watch television for an agreed-on time. The difference from the behavior modification techniques already described is that the parent and child engage in collective bargaining—comparable to that between unions and management. The child plays an active role in establishing the bargain and the standards by which his performance will be judged. In this instance it might include such items as bed made, clothes removed from floor and placed in hamper, towels hung up in bathroom, and so on. Likewise, the parents specify what they will do or permit when the contract is fully or partially fulfilled. Such a contract is typically made in writing, with each party clearly stating his obligations and the obligations of the other party, and it is signed by the child and each of the parents. It is called a contingency contract because the arrangement is, "If you do this, I will do that, and if I do that, you will do this." Each person's behavior is contingent—that is, dependent—on that of the other party to the contract. This kind of explicit bargaining has been used widely in dealing with hospitalized mental patients and is used by some therapists who practice behavioral family therapy. It has a ring of reasonableness about it, but its effectiveness has yet to be proven scientifically.

The above techniques may seem very mechanical to the parent who has diligently read books on child guidance and child-rearing. Most of these books stress that children misbehave because of deep-seated underlying problems, or lack of understanding of their own feelings. A valuable principle that has been provided by the operant therapists is that although these statements can be true, children are also mightily influenced by the consequences of their acts. Love is not enough. Understanding is not enough. If a child is to learn to behave desirably, his parents must become aware of what their own reactions are in response to his various kinds of acts.

A child may behave well without understanding or he may misbehave with full insight into what he is doing. The child may accurately describe himself as angry when he hits his baby sister. This is an interesting instance of the child's ability to comment on his own behavior. It is not helpful to his baby sister. For the child to be helped, and for the family to be helped, the child must learn to control his own behavior. If the child is to feel good about himself he may also have to learn about his own feelings. Helping the child understand himself and deal with his feelings will be discussed in the next session.

HELPFUL GENERAL PRINCIPLES AND TECHNIQUES

The general question of how parents should treat their children, of how they should relate to them in order to produce the healthiest possible psychological environment, has been the subject of numerous books. They carry a wealth of helpful advice for parents of all kinds of children, and no effort can be made here to review every approach that psychologists have found useful. However, I will briefly discuss certain general principles and techniques that are of special benefit to ADHD children as well as to children with no problems. When added to the previous discussion of basic procedures, they provide a good picture of psychological approaches that can be particularly useful in managing the ADHD child.

How to Criticize

No one likes criticism and children are no exception. Everyone can tolerate criticism best when it is specific, not generalized. For example, the spouse who arrives home from work and finds dinner not ready could respond with either of these two statements: "You are a disorganized person and never get anything done," or "I'm always starving after work and I'd really appreciate it if you could have dinner ready when I get home." The at-home spouse might not like either of the two statements but the second, being more specific and somewhat more understanding, is a lot easier to take. Similarly, an employer faced with a problem of chastising an employee who is late finishing a piece of work could select one of the following statements: "Jones, you are a lousy worker" or "Jones, I'd appreciate it in the future if you'd be faster getting me these reports." Again, the employee may not like *any* criticism, but the second version, being specific, is easier to swallow.

The same principle applies to criticism of children. When, for example, the ADHD child has just hit his baby sister for picking up his favorite toy, reducing her to a howling mass, the parent is likely to explode and say such things as: "Why must you be such a bad child?" "You're a terrible child and you're always making trouble!" "Can't you do anything right?" Reacting this way is understandable. Nevertheless, such an explosion is not helpful. If parents have thought about the problem areas in which improvement is wanted, they are in a far better position to criticize specifically. For example: "I do not like it when you eat with your hands— that is for small babies, not big children"; "Mommy gets upset when she asks you to clean up your room and you do not. Nobody likes to look at messy rooms. Please go back and clean it." In the examples given, the parent expresses anger— but for *specific* acts. It is perfectly all right and it is sensible for the parent to acknowledge feelings that a child knows are present. The child can see that the parent is angry. Denying what the child knows is not useful. But the parents must not allow their anger to take the form of criticizing the child as a whole. The parents must never call the child worthless or bad. When criticism is necessary, the parents should criticize the objectionable behavior and be as specific as possible.

How to Praise

Similarly, praise should be specific. Affectionate attention should be provided when the child is behaving desirably. If the child is eating nicely, say, "You are eating in a very grown-up fashion and that pleases me." If his baby sister is teasing him and he has resisted the urge to slug her, say, "I am very pleased that you can hold your temper even when Susie is making a pest of herself."

It is not very helpful to say, "You're a wonderful child," or to tell your spouse, "Jimmy has been just marvelous today." In addition to being ineffective in helping the child achieve self-control, such comments are likely to strike him as phony. All of us react to such comprehensive praise as false. We all know we have our good and bad points and that anybody who calls us "wonderful" is either trying to butter us up or is stupid. Children have the same reaction. Consider the TV talk show in which an actor is introduced as a "wonderful personality." That turns most of us off. We recognize it for the hokum it is. Thus, when you do praise children, praise them for the specific things that they have done that they know are good. Do not enlarge. Children recognize and appreciate honesty.

Recognizing the Child's Feelings

The general principle here is that children, like adults, need to be understood, especially by someone important to them.

Children have feelings. Recognizing those feelings and letting the child know that you recognize them often helps the child to feel better. It is extremely important, however, to realize that a parent can recognize a child's feelings and communicate that recognition without either criticizing or praising him. If the child is returning from his room, where he has been sent because of lack of control, the parent can help by saying something like "You must have felt that it is very difficult for a seven year old to always remember his table manners, and you must have been angry at Mommy for making you leave the table."

By recognizing and acknowledging feelings in a neutral way, the parent can make the child feel more comfortable.

Helping the Child Distinguish Between Feelings and Actions

The major principle here is that feelings can and should be expressed, even if they are bad. A part of the same principle is that feelings and actions are not the same thing. Children, like adults, often have feelings that "they should not"; they are sometimes envious, jealous, angry, resentful. All children have these feelings. In certain circumstances everyone has them. Children often feel guilty about having such feelings. They have learned that one should not be envious, jealous, angry, or resentful. It is very helpful if the parents, as discussed in the previous section, acknowledge to themselves that the child has such feelings (when he does) and let the child know that they (the parents) know. The parents must help the child distinguish between feelings (which are acceptable) and actions (which are not). Actions—that is, behavior—can be changed and shaped; feelings cannot be changed so directly and should not be treated as if they could be. If the child sees that his parents recognize and tolerate his feelings, his anxiety about having them may be relieved. His relief alone may often release enough steam so that the child will not act on his bad feelings. The child will feel less guilty if he knows that bad thoughts do not mean that he is bad and worthless in his parents' eyes. Since in the past he has acted in ways that have been considered unacceptable, he is likely to regard having comparable thoughts as equally reprehensible. The parents should repeatedly communicate to the child, directly and indirectly, that any bad thoughts that he might have are not terrible so long as he does not act on them. He will sometimes feel very angry with his baby sister; he should express such anger and his parents should help him express such angry feelings. He should not hit his baby sister. Parents should help the child understand the difference between thinking and doing.

The Technique of Labeling

One extremely important technique in helping the ADHD child to recognize and do something about his behavioral problems is labeling. Before the child can even begin to attempt to control his own behavior, he must know when he is doing something that is troublesome to others or hurtful to him. The catch is that many of these things are rather complicated. It is easy for a parent to tell a child, "When you lie down on the floor, scream, or pound your heels, that is a tantrum," and "Mommy will not talk to you until the tantrum is over, and if you cannot make it stop quickly, you will have to go to your room until it is over." A three year old can learn what a tantrum is. But some of the ADHD child's trouble-producing behaviors are more complex. For example, he may devise sophisticated techniques—and have a variety of them—for bugging his brother or sister. His father and mother cannot draw up a complete list of bugging behaviors. An enterprising, intelligent ADHD child can find multiple ways of annoying others. In order to help the child identify and recognize such behaviors, the parents should choose a code word. The code words I use are bugging and teasing. Every time the ADHD child bothers his brother or sister this way, the child is told, "You are teasing." After a few dozen repetitions—and parents will have many, many opportunities in the course of time—the child learns to recognize that a whole group of different things can be called teasing. It is no harder for the child to learn this than it is for him to learn that Great Danes, Dachshunds, and Chihuahuas are all dogs.

Once the child has learned what teasing is, the parents can expand the usefulness of the procedure by dealing with new occurrences in a different way. When Billy is pretending that he has lost his sister's doll, the parent can say, "Billy, what are you doing?" The intention now is to have him label his own behavior, which is a step toward taking more responsibility for it.

Labeling is a useful technique for several common problems, such as having trouble with attention or getting excited. Parents should actively look for and invent labels for the particular problems of their ADHD child that may lend themselves to this procedure. With repetitive labeling of this sort, parents of the ADHD child can generally help him to identify what he is doing. Remember that this is not easy. In *Games People Play*, Eric Berne spends a lot of time making up clever names for neurotic behaviors of adults. The reason the clever names are useful is that even adults, without the handicaps of ADHD, do not easily recognize the different ways they can be neurotic or just plain difficult. It is not surprising that an immature ten year old will have a hard time learning what is objectionable about his behavior.

Scientific investigation of the usefulness of teaching children to recognize their own troublesome behavior is in an early stage. Interestingly, Russian child psychologists have for some time been examining the ways in which language can help a child to control himself. They feel that self-labeling is the first step in self-control, and that the sooner the child learns to label what he is doing, the sooner he can learn to control himself. Although definitive evidence is not yet available, my clinical experience has impressed me with the usefulness of labeling as an additional parental technique.

THE MANAGEMENT OF COMMON PROBLEMS OF THE ADHD CHILD

The procedures, principles, and techniques described thus far refer to overall approaches to the ADHD child. In addition, I have some special suggestions that may be of help in managing a few specific common problems of these children.

Getting the Child's Attention

One of the ADHD child's major problems is paying attention. And one of the major problems of the parent of an ADHD child is getting the child's attention. If one wishes to communicate effectively with an ADHD child, one must use some special techniques. For example, often the parent will give a command to or make a request of an ADHD preschooler while the child's attention is elsewhere. In non-ADHD children such a parental request may catch the child's attention. In the case of the ADHD child, it usually does not. Even if the parent has the ADHD child's attention, the child may not wish to hear what the parent has to say and may place his hands over his ears or turn his head away. The following procedure should then be employed: the parent should take the ADHD child's head (or shoulders) gently in his (or her) hands and give the child the message. Then, to be sure that the child has received the message, the parent should ask the child what he was told, not in a punitive way but in a neutral tone. If the child does not know, the parent should make the statement again. Physical contact seems to play an important role in gaining the child's attention. When the message is given with the parent's hands placed on the child's shoulders, the child seems to pay better attention than he does when not touched.

Although these instructions have mentioned the pre-schooler, physical contact may still be useful with the older child as well. So is the procedure of asking the child what it was that he was told. Parents should remember that if they find themselves yelling in order to get the child's attention, something has gone wrong.

Rigidity

A characteristic of some ADHD children—although it can be seen in non-ADHD children as well—is rigidity. Rigid children are upset when their activities are interrupted or their routines changed. For example, they may become furious if they are stopped from playing with their toys so that they can be taken on a visit to Grandma's. Or they may begin screaming if the order of putting on their clothes is varied. One three-year-old ADHD child had a tantrum if the family drove to Grandma's house by a different route.

Rigidity sometimes disappears with age, but there are effective ways of dealing with it before that blessed time comes. The major principle is anticipation. Long before the break in routine occurs, the parent should repeatedly tell the child what is going to happen. For example, if the child is playing with his blocks and cars and the time to leave for Grandma's is two hours in the future, the parent should begin a countdown: "Billy, we will be visiting Grandma in two hours." Then, an hour later, "We will be leaving in one hour. It's time for you to put the trucks away." Next, "Billy, we are leaving for Grandma's in fifteen minutes. It's time to put the blocks away, change your clothes, and put your shoes on." With older children, to avoid repeated nagging, kitchen timers can be invaluable. Even before the child can tell time, he can recognize when the pointer is approaching the "O" that will start the bell. Rather than giving countdowns every morning for getting dressed to go to school, one can substitute the timer.

Similarly, considerable grief can often be avoided by discussing long-term changes before they occur. Repeated anticipatory talks about such matters as furniture moving, new sleeping arrangements, and altered school programs can frequently soften the blow for the rigid child. These procedures, of course, do not change the child's rigidity, but they lessen its unpleasant impact.

Spiraling Loss of Control

A very frequent problem of ADHD children, both as preschoolers and during the first few grades, is a spiraling loss of behavioral control. This refers to the child's becoming increasingly wild and behaving more and more immaturely once he is set off. For example, when guests come, the child may act in an attention-seeking manner, and as soon as he gets the attention, may react with foolish and noisy behavior that steadily worsens. After first telling the guests a story or showing them some of his models, he may begin to talk more loudly, start running around, and in some instances bounce off the walls. This may also happen in noisy or stimulating situations, such as at the supermarket or the circus.

How can this loss of control be handled? To begin with, it is helpful if parents learn to recognize the early symptoms of this behavioral breakdown. It is far easier to reverse such cycles shortly after they have started than when they are in full swing. When the parents recognize the symptoms of an impending behavior spiral, they should caution the child with a phrase that is always used when the child is excited—and here we see again the labeling technique in operation. Different parents use different phrases. Some parents will say, "You are getting too wild," while others might caution, "You are becoming overexcited." The important point is to label the same kind of behavior in the same way every time so that the child can learn what the parents mean by the special phrase. After the parent has identified the behavior, the child should be told to go to his own room and remain there until he has calmed down. If necessary, he should be taken to his room. Once he has calmed down, the child should receive no punishment but in fact should receive praise for having gotten control of himself and acting like a big boy. Then, in a nonaccusatory tone of voice, the parent should explain to the child what happened before and what caused the parent to label that behavior as wild or overexcited. In other words, parents should make sure that the child is praised (gets positive reinforcement) for acting quite grown-up, and that the child receives no extra attention—positive or negative—for being out of control.

Thus, the best thing to do about spiraling loss of control is to try to avoid it. To use a variation on an old cliché, parents should be ready with that invaluable ounce of prevention. They should learn to recognize the situations that trigger these spiraling reactions and either avoid them or remove the child as soon as possible from them.

Verbal Tantrums

One of the kinds of loss of control seen in both younger and older ADHD children is the verbal tantrum. Such behavior is probably more mature than breath-holding spells or down-on-the-floor kicking tantrums, but parents are not overjoyed at this kind of maturation. During the tantrum the child may talk (or yell) continuously, criticizing, blaming others, and denying responsibility. He may bring up not only trivial matters but also honest-to-goodness problems that exist in the family. These nonstop productions are limited only by his talkativeness and how his parents handle the problem. The natural reaction of most parents is to argue. The major advice I have is that a parent should not argue at all. A mutual screaming match solves nothing. While the child is having the tantrum, he should be told that matters will be discussed when he quiets down. If he is unable to quiet down, he should be placed in a time-out room, and only *after* he quiets down should the parent talk with the child about the real problem. Parents who frequently find themselves yelling can interpret that as a warning sign that they are doing something wrong—not bad, just ineffective.

Chores

Although particular chores have been used as examples in the preceding sections, I am giving special attention to the entire subject of getting the child to do routine, age-appropriate chores because it is one of the most common causes of friction between the school-age ADHD child and his parents. At first, nonperformance may be a result of forgetfulness and the child's inability to organize well. If the parents become angry and nag—and, except for a few saints, most become angry—the child may become increasingly stubborn and negative. This may lead to a snowballing of complaints by the parents and goldbricking by the child.

The best way to make sure that chores are done is as follows. First, list all the chores you want the child to do. Second, arrange them in order of importance ("1" next to the most important task, "2" next to the second most important task, and so on). Then, write down one or two of the most important chores on a homemade calendar and place this calendar in a conspicuous place, say, on the refrigerator. For example, if one chore is to set the table every other day (as sometimes happens when a brother or sister is also doing the same chore), the calendar should have the child's name listed on each day he is to perform it. If there are two chores involved, such as setting the table and clearing it, each should be listed separately on the day it is to be done (whether every day, on alternate days, or according to some other schedule).

Parents should avoid any disputes about what constitutes the chore by writing down its specific components. In setting the table, does one only have to place the silverware and dishes, or does one also have to bring the butter and milk from the refrigerator, and so forth? Assuming reasonably good parent-child relationships, many children will be compliant about chores if the requests are specific and structured enough.

If the child is resistant, the behavior modification principles I have mentioned should be employed. For example, parents could establish a rule saying that full payment of allowance will be made only if setting the table is done, without nagging, six times a week. With such a rule, if the chore is done only five times in a week, the child is docked in some mutually agreed-on way—such as receiving only five-sixths of his allowance.

After the most important chores are being done on a regular basis, the parents can move on to the next chore. Again, the calendar should be kept, and directions should be very clear and specific. Parents will avoid hassles if the rules are easy to understand and clear-cut. If they are not, the opportunity for legal arguments is much greater. And, as all parents know, most children are born lawyers.

Having the Child Take Responsibility for Himself

All parents hope that eventually the child will take responsibility for monitoring his own behavior. The procedure discussed under "Chores" illustrates one way of establishing a habit of responsibility. Here I will describe another method of encouraging responsibility. This example deals with another recurrent problem of the ADHD child—forgetting to bring his school assignments home, which means that he does not do his homework.

For this problem, I suggest that the child be given a small notebook in which he must write down *every day* after arriving home from school the work he actually accomplished at school and what was left undone in each subject that day.

If homework assignments are given, he should write down those assignments while he is in school, in the same book. It is his responsibility to write this information down. At the end of the week, the parent should contact the child's teacher to make sure that the child accurately recorded the completed work, the daily work that he did not finish in school, and the assigned homework. The trick with this technique is making the child responsible for telling on himself. I find that if the child reports accurately, he will be in a better position to proceed with the unfinished work and the homework and is more likely to complete both kinds of assignments after school. If the child fails to write the information down, he is docked part of his allowance or other privileges. In some instances, it may be better to start with a smaller allowance and reinforce the child by giving him an agreed-on bonus when he writes down the assignments correctly. After the child has mastered these tasks completely, the parents can often gradually withdraw the reinforcement and return to the usual allowance. After the notebook procedure has continued several weeks, the parents need only spot check with the teacher. However, as with most responsibilities expected of most ADHD children, the child should continue to use self-monitoring techniques long after his behavior is satisfactory. It is my impression that by really overdoing these techniques, parents can finally depend on the child to maintain some behavior patterns without such external supports.

Although this example involved school assignments, analogous procedures—with notebooks or calendars—can be worked out for such areas of the child's life as personal hygiene, grooming, music and dancing lessons, and so forth.

SPECIAL PSYCHOLOGICAL HELP FOR THE FAMILY AND CHILD

From time to time I have referred to the fact that in some families—either because of the presence of the ADHD child or for entirely different reasons—there will be much family stress and strain. These family difficulties cause problems for any child and they may cause greater problems for the ADHD child. If parents cannot agree between themselves about rules for their children, if they do not consistently reward or punish, if they criticize one child or favor another because of their own personal problems, they will create psychological difficulties for their children. Obviously, families with disturbances need professional help, regardless of whether they have an ADHD child, and this is the kind of situation in which help can be provided by psychiatrists, social workers, or psychologists. Any steps that will decrease difficulties within the family will be of special benefit to the ADHD child, since adjustment to even ordinary social demands is already difficult for him. Even if he responds well to medication, he may not respond to emotional stress as flexibly as a child who does not have the problems associated with ADHD.

Another form of specific psychological help that is *sometimes* useful for the ADHD child is psychotherapy, in which the child meets with a therapist, either individually or with other children in a group. The purposes of psychotherapy are to enable a child to recognize and understand his feelings and learn to deal with them appropriately. Psychotherapy, a very popular mode of treatment, has in the past been considered the best treatment for virtually all psychiatric difficulties both in adults and children. Currently, however, one of the major questions in adult and child psychiatry concerns the effectiveness of psychotherapy for particular problems. There are no data whatsoever supporting the usefulness of psychotherapy in the basic treatment of ADHD children. Nonetheless, many experienced psychiatrists have found that it is sometimes a useful auxiliary technique with some ADHD children. In my own experience it has been most useful with older ADHD children, especially those who have "engrafted" psychological disabilities on their temperamental ones. Many of the difficulties of these children concern interpersonal relations, and it is my impression that psychotherapy has proved useful with some of these children some of the time. These have generally been ADHD children who did not receive treatment with medication in their earlier years and as a result fell into the vicious circle of school and familial problems. They seem to have benefited from a relationship with a warm and impartial adult who was able to provide them with some understanding of their problems and help them in the construction of solutions to these problems.

Certainly individual psychotherapy is not the treatment of choice for most ADHD children. Unfortunately, the usefulness of medication and the other techniques discussed had not been recognized until fairly recently. In the past many ADHD children received psychotherapy, and for most of them it apparently was not helpful. Since it is a time-consuming and expensive procedure, it should only be used when there is a strong possibility that working with the child's special problems may be useful or when the child seems unresponsive to all other forms of treatment. This is certainly an area of dispute and some psychiatrists would undoubtedly disagree with me. All I can state is that I have seen dozens of ADHD children who have received psychotherapy, often for years, with no visible benefit, and who subsequently responded dramatically to treatment with medication. As I have repeatedly stated, the basis of most ADHD children's problems is physiological and must be dealt with physiologically—that is, with the aid of medication. Medication goes to the root of the problem. Psychotherapy may help to deal with some of the branches that, so to speak, have grown in the wrong direction. Many parents do not feel this way. I remember one very sophisticated mother whose seriously afflicted ADHD child responded dramatically to medication. At the first visit after medication had been started, the mother reported, "Tim is 100 percent better, Doctor. Now let's put him in psychotherapy and really get to the root of the problem."

Although psychotherapy is occasionally useful in some ADHD children, simpler measures should be employed first. If medication, educational remediation, and parental counseling fail to help the child as much as seems necessary, psychotherapy can be tried.

VACATIONS FOR THE PARENTS

Living with difficult children is difficult. The techniques I have discussed may make parents' lives easier, but their lives may still be much harder than those of most parents. For this reason I think it is very important for the parents of ADHD children to get away sometimes by themselves. (It is probably highly desirable for *all* parents. It is essential for the parents of ADHD children.) It is not a sign of intellectual, moral, or physical weakness for these parents to want a periodic vacation alone. ADHD children demand much attention, and caring for them can be physically, mentally, and emotionally exhausting. In addition, sometimes the parents' relationship suffers as a result of the tension surrounding the child's problems. The happiness and well-being of everyone should not be sacrificed for the good of the child with problems. Everyone deserves a piece of the pie. Thus, it is an excellent practice for parents to schedule regular time-out periods for themselves.

Obviously, such vacations pose practical problems. The ADHD child is often too much of a handful to deposit with unsuspecting relatives. If the community has an organization for parents of ADHD children, it might offer opportunities to share child care, with the parents taking turns at vacations without the children. Such trading has the advantage that all the adults involved are aware of the problems of the ADHD child and have some knowledge of how to handle them. This kind of trading off is not just of selfish value to the parents. If they are able to spend some time alone with each other and enjoy themselves, they may be more relaxed in handling their ADHD child when they return, which would benefit the child (and other children in the family as well). But whether or not this is the case, it is sufficient that the parents themselves will feel better.

EDUCATIONAL MANAGEMENT

■

ADHD children frequently experience academic difficulties that seem to arise from two major sources. First, most ADHD children are likely to have some problems in learning because of their distractibility, lack of stick-to-itiveness, readiness to give up, tendency to rush through things, and inability to discipline themselves (especially with respect to doing homework). *Some* ADHD children also have the specific learning problems in reading, spelling, and mathematics that are classified as developmental disorders and are called Learning Disorders (LD; see description in Chapter 2).

There are therefore two groups of ADHD children with learning problems: (1)those whose learning problems are secondary only to distractibility and inattentiveness; and (2)those whose learning difficulties are secondary to these inattention difficulties and also to Learning Disorders. Because of its effect on the child's overall organization and attentiveness, medication sometimes eliminates and frequently diminishes learning problems, particularly in the first group of children. However, even among those in whom the learning problems diminish with medication, additional educational assistance is often needed. Too often, by the time the ADHD child's academic problems are recognized and treated, he has failed to master basic material and has fallen behind in many subjects. Learning problems are cumulative, even in children of normal or above normal intelligence. Consequently, the child cannot compensate for his educational losses, despite improved functioning, unless remedial or "catch-up" tutoring is provided in those areas in which he has fallen behind. The problem of cumulative educational shortcomings is most severe in those ADHD children whose difficulties are first recognized in adolescence. They have often received social promotions and may be several grade levels behind in a number of subjects. Unfortunately, although medication may still be effective, appropriate educational facilities are often not available, and these children, frustrated and embarrassed by their poor academic showing, tend to give up.

The children with LD are another problem. Medicine *may* improve their attention span and stick-to-itiveness but it does not remedy their learning disorders. Scientific experiments have shown that stimulant medication is no more effective than an inactive placebo in facilitating learning in children with reading disorders. What is effective—to varying degrees—is special remedial education. However, although many people have investigated the teaching of "dyslexics," and people have recommended many different approaches with doctoral degrees in special education, there is no consensus about which children do best with which special education. Effective teaching can improve the reading and spelling performance of children with reading and spelling disorders, but with limits on the improvement that can be expected. Reading and spelling may continue to be problems as the child grows older, although the extent of the problem will vary, depending on the child's responsiveness, the nature of the teaching, the emphasis in the school, and the child's interests. For example, some private schools and a few public schools have been able to help children of normal intelligence with reading problems by the use of audiotaped material and oral tests.

Similarly, mathematics disorders—at least as far as arithmetic is involved—are now less of an academic handicap than they once were. The calculator has been an enormous help to those who have difficulty in doing complex addition, multiplication, and division. If the child can master columnar arrangement and the placement of the decimal point, he can solve the problems. Being calculator dependent may not be an asset, but it is certainly not a great liability.

Because many educators do not recognize ADHD children as a unique category, they frequently place such children in special educational classes, even though they have no specific learning problems. In addition, many children placed in these classes have both ADHD problems and learning difficulties. In both types a trial of medication is generally useful. To repeat, there is no way of predicting a child's response, and one may anticipate that some problems will disappear whereas others (including the learning ones) may remain. Any child who has been placed in a special class without a specific diagnosis of his difficulties should be carefully evaluated to see if he has ADHD problems and is therefore eligible for a trial of medication.

It may be useful to mention some educational approaches that have been tried but have not demonstrated effectiveness. A number of people had noticed that some children had both learning and coordination problems. (Approximately half of ADHD children do have some coordination difficulties.) These people reasoned, erroneously, that the learning problems were probably the result of the coordination problems. (Both are probably the result of a third factor.) They also believed that training in coordination might improve the learning difficulties. For this reason they prescribed exercises, involving either the whole body or the eyes. *At present there is no evidence whatsoever that coordination training will help the ADHD child's learning difficulties.* The same statement applies to specific treatment programs of eye exercises.

However, coordination training *may* help the ADHD child's coordination problems and ultimately his self-esteeem. The coordination difficulties from which many ADHD children suffer are frequently embarrassing or humiliating, particularly for boys. To be chosen last when teams are being picked and to be ridiculed for athletic inadequacy are blows to the ADHD boy's already shaky sense of self-esteem. There are programs in physical reeducation—not readily available—in which the children receive specific tutoring in motor tasks of increasing difficulty. My impression is that these programs sometimes improve the child's coordination and generally increase his self-confidence. If such programs are not available, the parent may help the poorly coordinated ADHD child by guiding him toward physical activity in which fine coordination presents less of a problem. As mentioned, many ADHD children have particular problems with hand-eye coordination and as a result are worse in such sports as baseball and tennis. Sometimes they encounter less difficulty in football—particularly in line play, where gross body movement is required—or in soccer. These children may often perform adequately or excellently in sports requiring large muscle control, such as running or swimming. Karate or tae kwan do are also good activities for the ADHD child; even though he may not do as well as the non-ADHD child, he can acquire skills that give him the novel feeling of being a "big man," a feeling that often considerably bolsters his self-esteem. Soccer, volleyball, and ballet would be good choices for the girl with ADHD.

SPECIAL PROBLEMS
OF ADOLESCENCE

■

The child whose ADHD is only discovered in adolescence poses several practical problems. The first is that he already has had years of unhappy experience as a result of his attention-deficit hyperactivity disorder. The second major problem is that adolescence is a time of rebellion for most children, ADHD or otherwise. Since the child is now increasingly independent, his cooperation in the treatment program is absolutely necessary. Furthermore, the behavioral techniques previously discussed are more useful with preadolescent children.

Most clinicians who treat many ADHD patients find that it is much easier to treat an adolescent who has been treated and followed since childhood than it is to work with an adolescent who has never been treated before. This is quite understandable if one thinks of some of the major psychological issues of adolescence. If an adolescent is diagnosed as having ADHD and if medication is recommended, think of what problems may follow. In general, the adolescent is not complaining himself. Like the ADHD child, he is brought to the doctor because he is not doing well and (probably) causing problems for others. But the adolescent feels that he is different—that he has different tastes, values, and wishes—and that treatment is being recommended not because he has a disorder but because he is not the way his parents would like him to be. Another issue is self-esteem. An adolescent's self-esteem is always shaky, and the ADHD adolescent's self-esteem is even worse. Learning that he may have to take medicine for a condition of which he was unaware (ADHD) can be another blow.

The difficulties in treating the adolescent for the first time are not insurmountable, but they do cause serious problems. If the adolescent can be convinced that the medication is something that is being done for him rather than to him, his cooperation can sometimes be obtained. Similarly, if he can be convinced that medication will give him more freedom by giving him more control of himself, he may be more willing to take it. Otherwise, he is likely to see medication as a chemical straitjacket employed by an oppressive adult world to control someone whose views differ. If he can be persuaded that medication will help him to control himself, he may accept its use. Unfortunately, without previous experience with the medication, he cannot know that he can still remain rebellious if he chooses to do so. He finds it difficult to understand that improved concentration will enable him to do better at studying subjects he is interested in—although he may still object to having to study some of the required parts of the curriculum.

Because of these problems in treating an ADHD adolescent for the first time, clinicians much prefer to treat ADHD symptoms when they become a problem in childhood. Treatment in childhood does not prevent symptoms in adolescence, but early experience with medication and with the therapist enables the child to understand that medication may help him and that the therapist can be a friend who is not an agent of his parents. If that child still requires medication in adolescence, he accepts it much more readily.

On the positive side, the adolescent is in a better position to understand and recognize the basis of his difficulties. This understanding, if it can be obtained, may balance out other problems. From a practical standpoint, helping the adolescent ADHD child generally requires the treating physician to spend more time in seeing the adolescent individually or with his family as part of family therapy.

If the ADHD adolescent has had serious learning problems, the situation may be critical. If he is five years behind in reading and spelling, school will be a nightmare. It is often difficult and sometimes impossible to convince such an adolescent that he is not a "retard." If he can be made to realize that he has reading problems that are not associated with intelligence and that he is not a moron, half the battle has been won. The second half is more difficult to accomplish. He must be entered in some kind of program in which his abilities will allow him to succeed and in which his disabilities will not seriously penalize him. If the public schools available to the youngster do not have the flexibility to help him explore the areas in which he might do well, it might be desirable for the parents to look for a specialized private school that offers more options.

SUMMARY

■

In capsular form I would like to repeat the major points of this chapter.

First, most ADHD children respond to medication. *All* ADHD children deserve a trial of medication since there is absolutely no way of predicting which children will respond well and which children will not. Sometimes medication alone is enough. Because the prescription of medication requires a doctor, a physician must always be involved in the treatment of the ADHD child.

Second, changes in the relationship between the parents and the ADHD child are almost always helpful. Understanding and establishment of firm, consistent, explicit, predictable rules are always useful. Frequently, these can be achieved with little or no professional intervention, yet sometimes the assistance of a psychiatrist, psychologist, or social worker may be helpful.

Third, some ADHD children need educational assistance. In many instances this will involve only remedial education, while in some cases it may mean special education. With such interventions, most ADHD children can be helped, often to a substantial degree. Not only will these forms of intervention diminish the present problems of ADHD children, but they will also often help to prevent future ones.

ILLUSTRATIVE CASE HISTORIES OF ADHD CHILDREN

■

Patient Name: **Arnold A**
Diagnosis: ADHD, Combined Type: Inattentiveness,
               Hyperactivity, Impulsivity

Arnold was a nine-year-old boy referred by his school public health nurse with the following complaints: "disruptive classroom behavior, a discipline problem at home. Outbursts of misbehavior—seems to lack self-control, especially when not under direct supervision of teacher (hits other children for no reason, rolls on the floor, jumps off chairs). Even under his teacher's direct supervision, he talks out, makes facial grimaces. He gets out of his seat frequently. Even during his 'quiet moments,' he seems tense; cracks his knuckles, plays with buttons on clothes, can't sit still. Has no close friends at school; seems to reject other childrens' attempts to make friends. He has above average ability, but not working up to that level now." The boy's behavior problems and academic problems had been aggravated by a family move and entrance into a new school. Reports from his previous school revealed, however, that Arnold had never been well adjusted; he had "spit, hit, and had temper tantrums . . . his behavior fluctuated drastically . . . sometimes he was moody and at other times exceptionally mean." By his mother's account, which his father tended to contradict, Arnold had always been very active, had been "always into things and on the go," had "no interest span," attentiveness, stick-to-itiveness, and had blown up easily and cried readily. He had marked sibling rivalry; his eleven-year-old brother had always been a model student and son.

When interviewed, he was a large, good-looking boy who talked openly and clearly, was not depressed or anxious, and had a good ability to relate. The first problem at referral was that his father had reacted to the referral with marked hostility, stating somewhat angrily that he had been similar as a child (and, although similar, had no problems) and had done pretty well.

The intake worker was initially unable to make Arnold's father less belligerent. He told Arnold's father the school's complaints about Arnold were not indirect criticisms of him as a parent. The worker, who was experienced and tactful, was eventually able to convince the father that he was concerned about how to help Arnold and was not trying to blame the parents for Arnold's problems. The parents were referred for couple counseling and Arnold for individual therapy. In the 1970s, this was the standard therapeutic approach. The therapist was a social worker who knew nothing of ADHD (then "hyperactivity") and missed the diagnosis—as would most non-child psychiatrists at the time. The usual interpretation was that childrens' problems were a consequence of how they were treated by their parents. The therapist, in the psychological jargon current at the time, interpreted his session with the parents as follows. "They [Arnold, his mother, and father] revealed a very pathological triangle with a very disturbed mother at the core. One can speculate that the interaction observed by this interviewer was typical of this family's interactions. The mother had rejected Arnold, and had labeled him as 'bad,' and the 'cause of all my problems.' Therefore, if he is removed (i.e., punished or locked up), things will be all right. The father is brought in by mother's excessive demands, since she is feeling overwhelmed and is dismayed at his being out of control (as his father is usually the instrument of Arnold's punishment). Arnold's reaction to mother's inability to maintain control appears to be his falling apart, impulsivity, and hyperactivity taking over, primarily at school. Hence, when mother is upset, his acting out behavior is unbearable both at home as well as at school. It is my opinion that Arnold is developing a chronic character disorder, and that without family intervention as well as therapy for him, specifically geared for their difficulties, therapy alone for him will be quite unsuccessful." The family therapy produced no benefit and Arnold was referred to a child psychiatrist who immediately diagnosed ADHD. He explained to the parents that the cause of the problems was largely biological and that they were not due to Arnold's meanness or willfulness or to a bad upbringing. They accepted his interpretation and both became more tolerant.

Following education of the parents and discussion of the therapeutic plan, Arnold started to take Dexedrine. Initially he was reported to be cranky, irritable, slowed down, moody, and to have insomnia. However, there was some slight improvement, and accordingly it was decided to increase the medication cautiously. Slowly increasing the dose over a period of several weeks allowed him to reach a dose that provided behavioral control without producing side effects. He returned to school, where his startled teacher reported that the hyperactive behavior had disappeared, that he had no difficulty with his peers, and that he attended to his studies. At home, his "temper" stopped entirely, discipline problems virtually disappeared, and he no longer fought with his brother.

An ironic and informative side effect of Arnold's successful treatment was the appearance of slight behavioral problems in his brother as Arnold improved. This phenomenon of one family member apparently becoming more ill as another becomes better is well recognized by family therapists and attributed by them to a need to maintain family balance. It is argued that one member's sickness was "serving a need for the family," and that *when this member's psychological adjustment improved, it was necessary for another member to become ill. There is another interpretation. In this family, what occurred was that the parents had previously not noticed the brother's comparatively minor difficulties until Arnold' conspicuous problems were ameliorated. When this happened, his older brother's minor problems became more visible. They began to discipline him for them and he reacted predictably, fighting more with his parents. The situation was explained to them and to the family in therapy, and the parents reduced their excessive expectations. The demands of the older brother, as well as his problems, gradually diminished.*

Patient Name: **Bobby B**
Diagnosis: ADHD, Oppositional Defiant Disorder,
                Clinical Depression

I first evaluated Bobby when he was fifteen years old. He had been referred by his parents because of continuing difficulties that had been unsuccessfully treated at a psychotherapeutically oriented child guidance clinic. The parents were concerned about their son's "continuing to do very badly in school . . . that has been true since kindergarten . . . his attitude is negativistic or just indifferent."

Bobby was the middle child of three children, all of whom had done poorly academically despite superior intelligence. His older sister, a sophomore in college, had obtained Bs and Cs in high school despite a high IQ. His nine-year-old sister had a full-scale IQ of 148 (which placed her well above the 99.9 percentile) and was getting low Bs. This sister was described as "unable to finish her work in school and unable to relate well to her peers." She was "wild, positive, domineering." On a scholastic aptitude test, Bobby placed above the 99th percentile ver-

bally and in the 87th percentile nonverbally. He obtained Cs and Ds in all his subjects at the time of this consultation.

The family background was most interesting. Bobby's father was an extremely bright, driven, self-made man, who had been raised in the backwoods of New England and was currently employed as a high-level computer executive. His school performance had been variable, and despite his ADHD he had obtained mediocre grades that he probably attributed to his brilliance. He "hyperfocused" and excelled in all aspects of computer subjects. His wife was an English-speaking ex-war bride, who had been chronically depressed for a period of several years. The parent's marital adjustment was poor. Where formerly they spent much time together, they now systematically avoided each other. The boy's father took every opportunity to take long business trips, while the mother kept herself at home. She had a large and close-knit family several thousand miles away, and had made no effort to develop close friends in this country.

The family was initially seen together, and the group meetings were sparkling. The mother emerged from her depression to talk intelligently and amusingly and joined in with a skill not to be expected in even a very clever depressed adult. Underlying the banter, his parents were worried and confused about their children's collective academic failure. Both had expressed their dissatisfaction with Bobby particularly, and he responded in kind. In their previous therapeutic experience, the family had been treated in a two-generation group. What the therapist perceived as the source of the problems was not clear, but the parents felt that he had repeatedly implied that they had been excessively demanding and had therefore caused their children's problems. It was quite clear that Bobby's performance (like his sibling's) was not in accordance with parental expectations. The parents were angry at the implication of the previous therapist that they had caused their children's troubles; they believed, rather, that they had merely reacted to them. As is usually the case after the fact, it was impossible to disentangle how many of the problems were initiated by the children and how much they were aggravated by the responses they produced in their parents. But there was no question that all three children showed ADHD symptoms at an early age and had academic problems from the time they entered school. There was a strong suspicion that the children would have had academic problems given any set of parents.

Bobby's developmental history was "classically" that of a child with ADHD of a combined type. He was "crying when born . . . and had problems from age two." He was described as hyperactive in early childhood, always on the go, and unable to sit still. He "habitually" destroyed toys and clothes, and had always been negativistic and excessively independent. He "antagonized other children who . . . wouldn't play with him." He was "almost kicked out of kindergarten," and had been maintaining a partial adjustment to authority ever since. He had been "destructive" in grade school, and had continually made inappropriate comments in class. As a school-aged child, he had clowned and talked loudly. As a brilliant adolescent, he baited his teachers, talked circles around many of them, and vented his proficient sarcasm on the slower ones; not surprisingly, he was very unpopular with them. He had never gotten into serious difficulty outside the home.

His parents reported in passing that he had been poorly coordinated all his life. Despite their efforts to teach him, he was unable to tie his shoes until he was ten years old. He was still a bad athlete in visual-motor sports, but had compensated by participating in track and swimming; he had wisely chosen sports in which many ADHD children succeed.

Bobby partially acknowledged that he was having difficulties, but attributed them—as did his family—to his superiority. He realized that others disliked him for his abilities, but he totally failed to see that he goaded them into hostility. His poor academic performance he attributed to a lack of interest, and, as a demonstration of his own academic abilities, he cited his performances outside of school. On interview, he revealed a side of himself that the parents did not recognize. He reported a mild chronic depression, a feeling that life was at best boring and often painful. He expressed other symptoms of clinical depression: guilt; frequent thoughts of death and occasional thoughts of suicide; sleep problems; low self-esteem and pessimism about his life and future; and he worried obsessively about the future.

I felt Bobby was an ADHD child whose initial ADHD symptoms had continued although changed with age, but who was suffering not only from a continuation of his previous difficulties, but also from psychological characteristics ingrained on the basis of these difficulties—and because of these he was in conflict with his parents. Finally, he was suffering from symptoms of a moderately severe biologically produced clinical depression. Because the depression seemed the predominant problem, he was begun on a trial of antidepressants, and within four weeks gradually began to experience an improvement in his mood. His ADHD symptoms—as expected—persisted and a course of Ritalin was introduced. His concentration improved, he quieted down, and stopped his angry argumentation with his teachers. He described himself as decreasingly boisterous, and manifested pride in what he perceived as his increasing ability to control his own behavior. Over the next several months his grades improved from Cs and Ds to Bs with two As. He and his parents received weekly psychotherapy, and then once every two weeks for a period of four months. During this time, he developed a new modus vivendi *with his parents. He acknowledged his father's domineeringness and his mother's depression and intrusiveness, agreed that these were defects that were unlikely to change, and began to accept their limitations. At the end of the six months, his school behavior and grades had improved, as had his family relations. The mother's depression had become more apparent, along with the boy's father increasing unwillingness to admit the now rather obvious mental illness in his wife and the probable biochemical problems in his children. He decided independently that he did not want his son treated with agents whose long-term effects were not known. Our scientific limitations were agreed with, but we mentioned to him that such possible dangers had not been demonstrated to be weighed against the present effects of discontinuing medication. The boy's father decided to discontinue both medications, and over the next several weeks Bobby's depression and boisterous school behavior returned, his grades declined, and his family problems reappeared. The boy's father became increasingly upset and depressed, withdrew from treatment, and refused to seek further treatment for either Bobby or his mother. Follow-up is not known.*

Patient Name: **Carl C**
Diagnosis: ADHD, Inattentive Type;
                Learning Disorder

Carl's mother brought him for evaluation when he was ten years old because of his behavior and learning problems in school. She reported that one of her other three boys (nine, twelve, and fourteen) had reading difficulties and spelling problems. The mother herself had rather serious reading difficulties as a child and even now, at age forty-one, had some slight persistent difficulties, which were not preventing her from getting her Ph.D. in social work.

The boy himself had an interesting history. His development was somewhat slow; he walked at one and a half years; he spoke in sentences at about three years. The parents had considered him quiet as a baby and perhaps somewhat fidgety as a toddler. Of his attention span, the mother reported, "If he is interested, he is there until it is completely done." The parents reported that he was unassertive socially. In preschool he was shy. Having entered nursery school at age four, he refused to talk and began again only when he was five. "He forms friends slowly . . . he doesn't fight . . . he is initially ill at ease with new children . . . the other children in my family are even less sociable." (Both parents describe themselves as having been shy during childhood, and both presented a picture of well-adjusted introversion.) The school complaints had been typical; short attention span, inability to complete work, and daydreaming in class. His IQ was normal, and he was reported to be very dexterous manually. Achievement tests revealed reading and spelling performance of a normal seven year old; that is, he was two years behind his predicted level of functioning and had a learning disorder. The mother was informed about the learning disorder, the school contacted, and arrangements made for receiving remedial help because of his problems with inattention and distractibility. The second part of the treatment was to give him a trial of stimulant drugs. His mother reported that the combined approach was very successful. Treatment had been "marvelous," with a total disappearance of his academic difficulties in school and an unasked-for improvement in his behavior at home. Although the mother had previously not complained of the behavior at home, she realized that when he was off medication in the summer, his behavior had reverted to its previous status, which had been less good than she had remembered. On the medication, his shyness lessened and he became more popular. The boy refers to Dexedrine as his "magic pills," and he never failed to remind his mother to give them to him on those rare occasions when she forgot. With continuing administration of medication and special education, his reading and spelling improved, although he still remained one to one and a half years behind the level predicted for his degree of intelligence.

He was maintained on medication, did adequately throughout high school, and elected—probably wisely on the basis of his learning disorders—to learn a trade. He has applied to a local vocational college for training as an automobile mechanic.

Patient Name: **Donald D**
Diagnosis: ADHD, Combined Type with some
                Conduct Disorder Problems;
                Learning Disorders

Donald was a fourteen-year-old boy referred to a child guidance center by the Juvenile Court. The court had become involved when the boy had been discovered repeatedly stealing small sums of money from the mother of a friend; he had used the money to make small purchases, not in any particular meaningful way (e.g., he did not use the money to "buy" friends). He had not begun stealing in response to any readily discernible change in his family fortunes, either financial or psychological. The court had apparently considered a psychiatric referral because the mother had stated that Donald had manifested other psychological difficulties as well.

At the time of referral, he was in the ninth grade, where he was getting Cs and Ds. This was representative of his past performance; he had never failed, but had obtained barely passing grades throughout his school history. At school, he apparently ingratiated himself with teachers, and only his mathematics teacher commented on Donald's inattentiveness, difficulty concentrating, and poor peer relations. His other teachers were impressed with the seeming psychological problems of his home life. One teacher indicated that Donald "had some concerns over his relationship with his step-dad. He has told me that there is a lot of disagreement between him and his step-dad. I think something important may be going on."

The mother indicated that at home there was indeed "something going on with his step-dad." Donald's father had died five years previously in an automobile accident. This was reported to have been an exceedingly traumatic event for the boy, who learned of his father's death on television before the family had been informed. Donald had been his father's favorite, and his mother—perhaps with a touch of jealousy—felt that Donald had always been overindulged and insufficiently disciplined. Most of his father's failings were "rectified" when the boy's mother had remarried one and a half years following his father's death. The boy's stepfather was rigid, hot tempered, and (the mother felt) "perhaps a little bit violent . . . so I'm afraid to interfere . . . particularly when he has been drinking." The stepfather had been increasingly upset by the boy's close ties with his mother, his poor school performance, and his "instigating" the younger children into various acts of misbehavior.

When interviewed, the boy was a good-looking, friendly, warm, open, sad child who was rather vague about the reason for his appearance at the court or clinic. He described his stepfather's jealousy of the close relationship between him and his mother. He stated that his relationship with his mother had been intensified by the feelings of being unloved by his stepfather. The boy was so warm and appealing, and he related so well, that it made the interviewer worry that he might be being manipulated in the manner of some conduct-disordered children.

Donald had four siblings, the oldest of whom was married and out of the home. An older brother was also getting along poorly with his stepfather; the younger children, both girls, were not. It seemed very clear to all mental health parties concerned that many of the boy's problems were secondary to a two-generation family triangle, which had been aggravated—as if often the case—by the presence of a stepparent.

Relevant aspects of Donald's past history were as follows: "as a baby and toddler, he had been very restless ... he always had to have something to do ... he was never able to sit still ... he had tons of nervous energy ... he couldn't sit still with reading ... he never sat for a moment in front of the TV." The mother described a low frustration tolerance, an extremely short attention span, and marked clumsiness, which in earlier days had resulted in his habitually breaking things and in later life had made him a conspicuously poor athlete. In regard to his peer relationships, his mother said that he was "never shy ... he has always been forward enough ... but he loses friends ... he never has any close friends ... he likes younger children he can boss around." At school, his marks had been at best Cs, and in the upper grades he had usually come home without his books, claiming that there had been no homework. On occasions when he brought work home, he failed to do it. His mother stated that his major problem was "a failure to learn to read right ... he is like his sister ... he can't grasp and retain, they say."

IQ tests showed him to be of normal intelligence, while his achievement tests found him to be three years behind in reading, spelling, and arithmetic, thus qualifying for learning disorders in these areas.

The mother was unable to explain why Donald's bio-

logical father had preferred the boy to his older brother, but stated that he always had. He felt that as a result Donald had learned to "take advantage of people and use them . . . he plays on their sympathy." She felt that the boy had little ability to discipline himself, that he failed to learn by discipline at home, but had learned to blame others for his own problems. The mother described increasing difficulties with her second husband, whom she blamed for aggravating the boy's problems. She felt that this husband was probably right but "too strong," and felt an increased need to take the part of her son.

Donald appeared to be an ADHD child, with learning disorders and the beginnings of antisocial characteristics. It was felt that his problems had been aggravated by the handling of both fathers. With limited expectations (because of the clear-cut antisocial behavior), he was begun on Ritalin with caution, and the dose was gradually increased. His mother stated that on the medication he became quieter, more tractable, easier to talk to (in which judgment his probation officer concurred), and his grades improved at school, most Ds having been advanced to Cs. She still felt that the boy continued to be unusually demanding of attention and fearful of being "left out." Donald described feeling "pretty good," and stated that medicine had made his head "feel clearer" so that he could concentrate much better ("I feel a lot more relaxed"). His school reported improved academic performance—increased attention, better concentration, decreased daydreaming, decreased stubbornness with a teacher—and improved peer relations (his fighting had diminished considerably). His probation was terminated after a year. His mother reported no antisocial behavior, and although I wanted to get the stepfather into therapy to lessen the friction between him and Donald, I was unable to do so. He continued to do well on medication for the next two years, and then he and his family moved away. I do not know if he continued to receive medication, and have no knowledge about the continuation of his antisocial symptoms.

Patient Name: **Elaine E**
Diagnosis: ADHD, Primarily Inattentive Type

Elaine was brought to a child guidance clinic when she was eight years old. She presented no behavioral problems whatsoever, either at home or school, but was getting poor grades. She had always seemed to be a bright child, an observation that was verified by intelligence testing, but she was one to one and a half years behind in reading and spelling. Her mother described her as having been a quiet child, inclined to daydream, who would amuse herself for hours. As a preschooler, she loved to be read to, or, specifically, she liked certain books that she would listen to over and over. If the story was uninteresting, she rapidly lost attention. Temperamentally, she was very much like her father, who had been a quiet, "average" child. He had gone to high school, college, and law school at a low B level of functioning and had become an associate in his father's law firm. He, like his brother, was somewhat dreamy, conscientious, moderately effective, but not an energized go-getter. He felt more comfortable with Elaine's school problems than her mother did.

Elaine represented a type of ADHD child whose problems have been neglected, at least until recently. This is the ADHD child whose primary problems are in inattention, who will not focus on something he or she is uninterested in. The school problem is that the child's attention is not under "social control." She would not attend to subjects that she feels are particularly boring, and which primary education teaches by rote. (For some reason the non-ADHD child can attend when asked to; the ADHD child cannot.) Because these children are not dis-

*ruptive in school, they are frequently overlooked. Elaine
was such a child.*

*She was begun on treatment with Dexedrine and her
grades improved quickly. Concentration improved, distractibility decreased, and daydreaming almost stopped.
She remained a quiet, slightly withdrawn child, but her
academic performance improved and she became somewhat more extroverted.*

*Elaine is currently twelve years of age, and still requires
and responds to treatment with Dexedrine. Her grades are
average and she presents no behavioral problems.*

Patient Name: ***Fred F***
Diagnosis: ADHD, Combined Type: Inattentiveness/
                  Hyperactivity/Impulsivity/
                  Oppositional Defiant Disorder and
                  early Conduct Disorder

*Fred was eight years old when he was brought to a child
guidance clinic, where his mother recounted a "classic"
history of ADHD. She stated that he had been very active
from the time of birth, had shown rapid motor development, walking under a year, and had as a toddler manifested extremely destructive behavior that was not mali-
cious: the boy was good-natured, but was always a "bull
in a china shop," breaking toys and lamps, and wearing
out his clothes at a prodigious rate. As a toddler and pre-
schooler, he had been impossible to discipline. He inevitably—and good-naturedly—"forgot," although when
carefully supervised he would willingly perform a task.
He was extremely outgoing and, until the third grade, had
adjusted well with teachers and peers. Despite his non-
compliance, his genuine good nature had prevented anyone from becoming seriously resentful of the boy. His parents had been able to tolerate his behavior, and consulted
the clinic only because Fred was beginning to have aca-*

demic difficulty in school and to manifest antisocial behavior, stealing small amounts of money from his
mother's purse, and small articles from stores. Fred was
a good-looking, friendly, obviously intelligent boy, and
when interviewed with his parents, we discussed their
concerns about him and their reactions to him; he acknowledged some difficulty, and while not acknowledging his problems, did not deny them either. He had a diagnosis of ADHD, Oppositional Defiant Disorder, and
beginning Conduct Disorder.

The parents were counseled, and the boy was begun on
drug therapy. Large doses of Dexadrine and Ritalin proved
ineffective. The parents were given education in techniques of behavioral management, which reduced his
symptoms somewhat. Over the six years of follow-up, his
symptoms improved somewhat. Since junior high school,
his grades and behavior both deteriorated. This is typical
of untreated ADHD children, or children who (like Fred)
did not respond to therapy. His academic problems were
intensified by no longer having a teacher who knew him,
who was aware of his strengths and weaknesses, and who
was able to closely monitor his progress. The problem is
worsened in middle and secondary school because the
child now becomes responsible not only for moving from
class to class, but for obtaining assignments, showing in-
itiative, working on assignments, and returning them.
Children who do not respond to medication will experience increasing school pressures and increasing failure.
Fred began to lose interest and motivation and to "hang
out" with the other children who were beginning to fail
academically. Like other such children, Fred began to engage in antisocial activities. When combined with the
"normal" rebelliousness of adolescence, these behaviors
can lead to substance abuse, and, ultimately, to failing in
school. ADHD children like Fred are fairly common, and
better therapeutic techniques are necessary to treat them.

Patient Name: *George G*
Diagnosis: ADHD, Combined Type

George was first seen when he was ten years old. His mother stated that George had multiple problems: "he has no impulse control, he's aggressive with other children . . . when he starts things he can't stop . . . (he) lies about anything and everything, plays with matches, (is) attracted to dangerous things (e.g., the oven), does poorly at school, can't concentrate, must touch everything, and takes things apart."

His problems may possibly have been due to slight brain injury. His medical history included the following: he was two months premature; his birth weight was 3 lbs 10 oz; he was placed in an incubator for six days and was kept in the hospital for six weeks.

George had received his first psychiatric evaluation when he was six and in the first grade, and his parents had been in individual and couple therapy for three years. They stated that the problems had not been helped, and that, if anything, they had gradually become worse. When interviewed, George was of average intelligence, friendly, and showed some minor neurological symptoms on neurological examination; these supported the possibility that his problems had not been caused by genetics but by damage during his early development in the womb. After the rationale of the treatment was explained to the parents, he was begun on a trial of Dexedrine. His very surprised mother reported few problems after one week, and when he was seen two weeks later she reported that he was doing "excellently in school" and had been very pleasant at home. A month later she reported with further surprise that "he was beginning to make friends . . . he is in on time . . . he does what he is told . . . children come to the house for him . . . he has never been so good for so long in his whole life before." The school reported that

"George's behavioral change has been a grand improvement. He does not seem as flighty as he appeared during our first semester. His frustration level has been reduced to a level that allows for normal productive days in the classroom. He does now sit and work attentively for a greater length of time than he previously was able to do; his mood has come to be one of a receptive nature to all guidelines of an academic and disciplinary nature. He seems to be more valued as a friend than before. Children now seek his opinion and respect his worth as part of a class." He remained on medication through high school. Trial discontinuations resulted in decreased concentration, decreased ability to function well at school, and mood swings. He moved away for college, and his family moved as well. His mother reported that he had continued to take medication while at college, also that he was doing reasonably well academically, getting Bs, and was having no problem with social adjustment.

6

Attention-Deficit Hyperactivity Disorder in Adults

■

When the previous edition of this book appeared in 1987, I advanced the reasons why I believed that ADHD in adulthood was common, diagnosable, and treatable. Those reasons were based on research that my collaborators, Drs. Frederick Reimherr and David Wood, and I had conducted (and published on) since 1976. We undertook controlled experiments on the effects of various drug treatments on approximately 200 patients whom we diagnosed as ADHD children "grown up"—that is, adults with continuing problems of ADHD. In addition, we conducted experiments on metabolism and drug responsivity in an effort to elucidate the mechanisms of the presumed underlying chemical abnormalities in nearly one hundred patients with ADHD, and we treated scores of patients clinically. Our experience is therefore based on the treatment of several hundred ADHD adults. (It has been a tremendous scientific advantage to be able to work with adults. They can provide information about the inner experience of being ADHD—something children cannot do—and we have been able to learn about the feelings, reactions, and lives of ADHD adults in a way we never could from our studies of children. We can ask them to give informed consent to allow us to conduct nontherapeutic experiments—something one cannot do with children who cannot give truly informed consent.) Reports on our work have been judged by editorial boards consisting of experts in the field, were published in scientific journals, and have convinced many other clinicians that ADHD may indeed persist in adults in their thirties, forties, and fifties, and that in many instances adults with ADHD respond to stimulant medication in a way similar to children with ADHD.

At the time we began, most child psychiatrists believed that ADHD diminished in adolescence and disappeared in adulthood. Since then other investigators have explored the development of ADHD children into adolescence and adulthood. As I discussed in Chapter 4, probably one-third to two-thirds of ADHD children continue to have problems in adult life, and in one-half of them the symptoms are marked enough to interfere with their functioning as students, workers, partners, or parents. A view that was held in the past was that the reaction of ADHD children to stimulant medication was "paradoxical." Whereas stimulants usually produce euphoria and excitement in adults, they seemed to result in quietness and settling down in ADHD children. It is not clear whether this same effect is produced in normal children because no one has given stimulant drugs to non-ADHD children over a period of weeks or months. However, when non-ADHD children with learning disorders are given stimulant drugs such as Ritalin, they do not calm down but instead often become anxious, irritable, and driven. Twenty years ago the common belief was that, as ADHD children outgrew the problems during adolescence, their paradoxical response went away, and then, as older adolescents and adults, they responded to stimulant medication in the normal way by becoming excited, stimulated, and euphoric.

Reports of clinicians who noticed that adults with apparent ADHD could benefit from stimulant medication were generally neglected. Why? In psychiatry, beliefs arise either because many practicing clinicians observe the same phenomena over and over or because scientific studies demonstrate and affirm the clinician's observations. Twenty years ago clinicians who treated ADHD in childhood were just beginning to observe its course systematically, and they frequently disagreed. Psychiatry and child psychiatry have made substantial advances in the past twenty years, and what was then a matter of clinical observation is currently being confirmed scientifically. Others have replicated our drug studies and found that ADHD adults respond to stimulant medication in the same ("paradoxical") way that ADHD children do.

As I have discussed in Chapter 4, considerable further evidence has now accumulated indicating that ADHD frequently persists into adolescence and into the mid-twenties. Recent studies of ADHD in adults have found the symptoms present in still older people. In our last major study of over 100 patients with ADHD, the average patient age was thirty-nine.

In the previous edition of this book, I also wrote that two questions remained. Both have now been tentatively answered. The first was: How common is ADHD in adults? Depending on how ADHD in childhood is diagnosed, somewhere between 3 and 10 percent of preadolescent children suffer from the disorder. The follow-up studies I have discussed find that about one-third to two-thirds of former ADHD children have continuing ADHD problems. If we base our adult figures on the 3 percent rate of childhood ADHD, then 1 to 3 percent of adults would have continuing ADHD problems. But if the figure for ADHD in childhood is 10 percent, as many as 4 to 5 percent of adults may have continuing and impairing symptoms of ADHD. From a practical standpoint, psychiatrists conducting diagnostic evaluations of the parents of ADHD children find such symptoms very frequently. The second question was: What are the distinguishing features of ADHD in adulthood? In our own research, we have listed the symptoms we believe are present in adults with ADHD. Before I describe them, I want to emphasize that methods such as we have employed must be confirmed by other psychiatric researchers before they can be widely accepted. We have employed all the techniques customarily used to reduce chance of self-deceit—that is, to reduce the chances of our persuading ourselves that what we expect to find is true. However, the help of other psychiatric researchers is needed not only to confirm our methods but also to aid in independently identifying the symptoms of ADHD in adults. Their help is particularly necessary for sorting out ADHD symptoms that are very similar to and can be confused with biological (clinical or chemical) depression.

What was novel twenty years ago is accepted scientific knowledge today. ADHD in adults has gone from being an obscure diagnosis to being (it sometimes seems) the diagnosis of the decade. The problem facing psychiatrists now is not to overdiagnose ADHD.

Even though this is a book that focuses on ADHD in children, I am including a section on ADHD in adults because it may shed light on the ADHD child's later development, because it may be applicable to the parents reading this book, because we have done scientific research on nearly 300 patients that is not generally known by laypersons, and because not much popular writing based on research has been published on the subject. Since ADHD clearly runs in families, the parents of the children and adolescents discussed are more likely to have had ADHD in childhood—and adulthood—than people in general. My hope is that adults reading this book—not necessarily just the parents of ADHD children—who recognize in themselves the signs and symptoms indicated below may be motivated to receive formal evaluation for possible treatment. I would like to educate adult patients with ADHD on how they can be treated most effectively.

THE SYMPTOMS OF ADHD
IN ADULTS

■

OVERT SYMPTOMS

The symptoms of ADHD in adults that I am going to discuss are those that my colleagues at the University of Utah and I used as we explored this disorder. We discovered these symptoms by talking to adults whose parents had been contacted and whom we could retrospectively diagnose as having had ADHD in childhood. We then questioned these adults and their partners about the symptoms they experienced and the maladaptive behavior they exhibited. The official *Diagnostic and Statistical Manual* employed by the American Psychiatric Association cites the behaviors in ADHD children observed by others (so-called "signs"), not the internal experiences (symptoms) of the children, as criteria for diagnosing ADHD. Children are generally unable to articulate or describe their inner life. But many adults can provide us with a detailed account of the emotional and intellectual response that an ADHD adult experiences. Thus, these adults gave us the first full reports from within the disorder and taught us what it feels like to be ADHD, not simply what it looks like to an outside observer. Taken together, the symptoms are referred to as the Utah Criteria. We devised the Utah Criteria to describe symptoms that are frequently seen in—and cause severe problems for—ADHD adults, but that are not seen in ADHD children. The symptoms in children are formally listed in the *Diagnostic and Statistical Manual*, 4th edition (known as DSM-IV), and are reproduced in the Appendix. As they apply to children, they were discussed in Chapter 2.

In our early studies, when the diagnoses of ADHD in adults was not widely accepted, we restricted the studies to adults who had the most typical symptoms: *both* attention deficits *and* hyperactivity. See the Appendix for more information on ADHD, Combined Type. We wanted to begin our studies with the most clear-cut cases of ADHD. We have subsequently diagnosed and treated individuals whose problems were predominantly in attention and had no symptoms of hyperactivity, either as children or adults. Although many of these patients show a good response to treatment with medication, the diagnoses must be made with great care because attention problems are seen in many other types of psychiatric disorder and do not respond to stimulants. Indeed, they may even worsen when treated by stimulants. Again, it is important to emphasize that our diagnostic methods are still being worked out and that neither we nor other researchers know exactly how much many of them should be present for a definite diagnosis.

The first requirement for having a diagnosis of ADHD in adulthood is that the person *must* have had ADHD in childhood. That is, beginning before the age of seven, the child had the persistent symptoms of inattentiveness and/or hyperactive/impulsive behavior discussed below. ADHD does not develop in adults who did not have it in childhood.

Most adults have sketchy memories of their childhood and cannot remember whether or not they had the specific symptoms of ADHD. If the adult cannot remember his or her childhood behavior in detail, good answers may often be found from the adult's "rearing" figure—usually the mother— by asking her about the specific symptoms of childhood ADHD. How to do this—what should be asked—will be discussed in the summary of the Utah Criteria in the Appendix.

However, and this is a big however, children with other psychiatric problems may have the same problems of inattentiveness, impulsivity, or hyperactivity. Therefore, even if an adult behaved this way as a child, a diagnosis of ADHD can be made only if those childhood symptoms clearly were not produced by any other form of psychiatric disorder.

The following problems are those we have found to be experienced by the ADHD adults we studied. Because the study of ADHD in adults is comparatively recent, ideas about the symptoms themselves—for example, which ones *must* be present to make the diagnosis and which are *frequently found but not necessary*—are still changing. According to the official DSM-IV diagnostic criteria (see the Appendix), the child must have inattention and/or impulsivity-hyperactivity. Our criteria for the diagnosis of ADHD in adults, the Utah Criteria, also follow. They consist of hyperactivity and inattentiveness and two of the five additional symptoms discussed below.

Attention Problems

Our patients experience the same sorts of problems with *attentiveness* that we observe in ADHD children. They are often able to concentrate on material that interests them but not on what doesn't. This is true even if the uninteresting things are important. They could not concentrate on fractions as a child. They cannot concentrate on an income tax form as adults. When this problem is severe, they may find it very difficult to read. The inattentiveness often causes difficulties at college, at work, and in other situations in which attention is required for learning. The symptom is often present socially as well, and frequently they are unable to keep their mind on conversations. They do not hear what their spouse said, and, as I will mention later, they impulsively reply before she is finished or finish her sentence for her. There is no conversational give-and-take. The same inattentiveness causes problems when they are talking with a group of people. They hear only part of what is said. They miss the drift of the conversation so that when they talk—often interrupting—they have missed the point and talk about something unrelated. The others may wonder where the ADHD adult is "coming from" and give him surprised looks. He is not wanted as a social participant. All psychiatrists working with couples have many times heard the complaint that the spouse does not listen; it is a usual complaint from the spouse of the ADHD adult. Thus, another consequence of the inattentiveness can be disturbed social relationships.

In addition to inattentiveness, patients often complain of *distractibility*. Their train of thought or their activities are interrupted by irrelevant things. They forget where they were or fail to complete their task. One woman, a historian, reported that the following kinds of experiences kept her from working when she sat down in her study: first she would hear the refrigerator go on; next she would respond to the cat coming through the cat door; then she would be disturbed by the continuing rustling of leaves on the roof. Being constantly disturbed by such stimuli made writing extremely difficult. When she was later treated with stimulant medication, she reported that not only could she focus on her work but she also was able to shut out such distracting noises.

Hyperactivity

Although hyperactivity is not necessary for the diagnosis of ADHD in childhood, and often disappears as the child grows older, we have studied only those individuals who were hyperactive as children. In this early phase of the investigation of adult ADHD we have used this narrow definition because we wanted to study the most definite—and perhaps extreme—cases. We have done this because we wanted to reduce the risk of studying and treating people whose symptoms look like those of ADHD but in fact are produced by other disorders.

However, we have found that hyperactivity, if present in childhood, usually does persist. When hyperactivity continues into adult life, it takes a somewhat different form than in childhood. Of course, our adults do not go running around classrooms anymore, but they are still frequently out of their seats. Often they report nervousness. What they mean is not that they are anxious or worrying but that they grow impatient when sedentary activities are prolonged. They find it difficult to remain seated while watching a movie or TV, reading a newspaper, or studying at college. They feel a strong urge to get up and walk around. They feel more comfortable while being on the go, and they are uncomfortable when forced to be inactive. Some patients report that they have an increased ability to sit still if they have first performed vigorous activity. One young woman reported that in high school she could concentrate on her homework for only ten or fifteen minutes at a time, but that she could study longer if she first expended a lot of physical energy. In her case this involved taking an elevator down to the first floor and then running up the twelve flights of stairs to her apartment. After expending this energy, she could concentrate for a full half-hour. Many of our patients are fidgeters. We have had the repeated experience of identifying a new patient in the waiting room as the one continuously drumming on the arm of a chair, as the one tapping his heel, or the one jiggling a crossed leg. During our diagnostic interviews we often find such patients squirming in the chair, tapping their feet, playing with their hands, or picking at their face and hair.

Impulsivity

Our patients describe difficulties in self-control. They have a tendency to act first and think second. They have difficulty tolerating frustration and often act to relieve that frustration instead of thinking things through carefully. They tend to do things on the spur of the moment and regret their actions later. They do not like postponing decisions and, because they do not think things out, they often do not anticipate fairly obvious consequences of their actions. Socially, like ADHD children, they tend to interrupt when other people are talking.

The negative consequences of impulsivity are greater for

adults than for children. Whereas running on the playground may result only in a teacher's reprimand, reckless speeding or gambling often has more serious consequences. The combination of impulsive decision-making and a short fuse (discussed below) causes some ADHD adults to be aggressive and dangerous drivers. ADHD adults are more likely to have accidents, license suspensions, and speeding tickets. Looking only at present pleasure and avoiding thoughts of future pain, adults with ADHD can be impulsive buyers (aided and abetted by credit cards), initiators of foolish business activities, and participants in short-lived romances and marriages. One unsubtle instance of impulsivity occurred in our pemoline study. A patient asked me to compliment him because "I'm getting married." When I said, "I didn't even know there was anybody on the scene," he replied, "There wasn't—we've only known each other for three days." I did compliment him, and then realized he had probably recruited another subject—his wife-to-be.

Mood Swings

Another area in which difficulties are often seen is mood. Our ADHD patients describe problems with mood that frequently go back as far as they can remember, often before adolescence. What they tell us is that their mood changes frequently. They describe being very reactive—that is, they tend to become depressed much more readily and to a greater degree than other people when they encounter frustration, loss, or defeat. They also tend to shift in the opposite direction. They will describe becoming excited and over-stimulated when things go well, and they distinguish this feeling from genuine happiness. It seems to be the adult equivalent of the overexcitement one sees in ADHD children in stimulating environments, such as the supermarket or the circus. As they get older, the excited periods seem to occur less often. Their moods come and go quickly. Their downs can be relieved by a change in circumstances. Our patients have also told us that their moods frequently shift by themselves for no apparent reason. Their ups and downs last a few hours or at most a few days. Some ADHD patients have described their mood fluctuation as resembling being on a roller coaster or moving up and down like a yo-yo. When a depressed mood lasts for a longer period, it is because the patients have "dug themselves into holes" in life. The depression is described as being "down," "bored," or "discontented"—and frequently patients distinguish it from sadness.

The mood problems of ADHD are different from those experienced by patients with other mood disorders, such as biological depression and manic-depression. Yet a patient may have both ADHD and another biologically produced psychiatric disorder, specifically, clinical depression and manic-depression. To provide an accurate diagnosis, the evaluating physician must be sufficiently experienced in working with psychiatric disorders in adults. Such a physician must question the patient who has ADHD mood problems about other mood problems that may exist at the same time and may require different treatment.

Unlike the depression associated with ADHD, biological depression can last day in and day out; patients may be depressed for weeks, months, or years. Also, the experience of biological depression is different. Patients with this kind of depression report that they lose enthusiasm, motivation, and derive no pleasure from things they used to enjoy: eating, watching television, making love, listening to music, doing their hobbies. In addition, patients with biological depression have changes in their sleep patterns, appetite, and energy level; they may have feelings of worthlessness or guilt and thoughts of death or suicide.

Similarly, the "highs" that the ADHD adult experiences are different from the elevation of mood seen in manic-depression. The ADHD adult's "ups" are described like the excitement we have seen in the ADHD child. The "ups" that the manic-depressive patient experiences, however, are more euphoria than excitement; they are described as "flying . . . being on cloud nine." During these euphoric periods the manic-depressive individual may experience *increased* self-esteem, a decrease in the need to sleep, a racing of thoughts, increased sexual activity, and serious and possibly self-destructive impulsive behavior.

Disorganization and Inability to Complete Tasks

Our patients describe difficulty in organizing their lives in both minor and major ways. They are disorganized in solving problems and structuring their time. They tell us that at home and at work they frequently move from one task to another before completing the first one. Because of such plan-lessness and shifting around, they often report that it takes them much longer than it should to complete projects. The kind of shifting they describe is not what we all adopt to avoid boredom (I'll read this book for an hour, then balance the checkbook, then prepare dinner). They recall having jumbled desks at school, and, if they are white-collar workers, they now have trouble setting priorities and finding what they need in their desks and files. One car salesman was not able to see why his wife was apoplectic about his failure to organize and why his boss was about to fire him because his sales records were incomplete for six months. One despairing husband of an ADHD woman described their refrigerator as having been taken over by a rich collection of bacterial and fungal life, apparently unnoticed by his wife. His wife, the co-parent of three "hyperactive" children, was a witty, lit-erate, absentminded professor, who had never mastered the art of household organization—or even sequentially button-ing her invariably stained white blouses. At home, ADHD adults may find it difficult to pay bills on time or to keep track of tools. If they continue with school, their efforts are hamstrung by the same disorganization they had as children.

One ADHD patient described, with horror and humor, her preparation for her eight-year-old son's birthday party. In the middle of washing the breakfast dishes she suddenly realized that she was giving a birthday party that afternoon. Before finishing the dishes she went out to get party favors, returned home, and then realized she had failed to buy the cake mix that was needed. Without prioritizing, she also remembered that a large load of laundry had to be done. She started to do that before completing the morning dishes or baking the birthday cake. By the time children began to arrive, she was completely frazzled. Another example is that of a man who started to panel his unfinished basement, but halfway through was struck with the thought that this was early summer and therefore a good time to stain the deck; before completing either of those tasks, he decided to grout the bathroom tiles, which had been in a poor state of repair for some time. A year later the basement was still uncompleted. A great deal of unorganized energy was inefficiently expended.

It is important, however, to distinguish this tendency to jump from one thing to another, which may be a facet of impulsivity, from a realistic response to the multiple pressures of a busy daily life. For example, a well-organized woman who has young children, is employed, and takes care of her own home often cannot complete all she would like to do in any one day, but this has no relation to ADHD. In contrast, the lack of ability to plan activities adequately is the characteristic that may be a symptom of ADHD in an adult.

Short and Hot Temper

During childhood, many but not all ADHD children are described as having a low boiling point or a short fuse. As children they may have had more than their share of temper tantrums and fights at school. The ADHD adults we have seen tend to have short-lived anger. They explode, but do not nurse anger or brood. With age, some have learned how to count to ten, while others have learned that for them the only effective technique for avoiding an explosion is to leave the scene. Temper outbursts sometimes produce the most serious problems patients have to face. Bad temper may cost them jobs, destroy personal relationships (including marriage), distance them from their children, and end friendships.

Most ADHD patients report that although their fuse is short, they calm down quickly—they do not nurse grudges. They often find it difficult to understand why, after their outburst, their spouse is then upset for hours or days. An extreme instance is that of an ADHD man who, in the midst of an argument with his wife, threw her *up*stairs; fortunately, she was not badly hurt. However, he was surprised that she did not feel romantically inclined that evening.

Low Stress Tolerance

Finally, we also see in the adults with ADHD an over-reactivity that is a hard attribute to measure but very important to our patients. They describe themselves as having a chronically thin skin. They become easily flustered, hassled, tense, or uptight. They perceive themselves as making mountains out of molehills and becoming readily distressed, and they frequently find themselves psychologically incapacitated by minor difficulties. Stress is often blamed for both physical and psychological disorders. Stress reduction is often suggested to relieve physical symptoms or lessen psychological problems. If stress reduction techniques, like meditation or aerobic activity, are successful, all is well and good. However, we tend to forget that a stress response is normal and functions in our lives all the time—physiologically and psychologically we are designed to contend with stress. The ADHD person's response to stress, however, is exaggerated and even inappropriate. Such a person could become equally upset over a facial pimple as over a broken leg. Overreacting to stress also increases a person's difficulties in solving problems, which makes a bad situation worse. It also produces a vicious circle: failure to solve problems increases tension, which in turn results in a decreased ability to solve problems, and patients may become overwhelmed and demoralized.

OTHER PROBLEMS

Having ADHD does not mean that the individual cannot have other biologically produced psychiatric disorders, such as biological depression, as discussed in the section on mood problems. Some ADHD patients have an accompanying persistent anxiety different from the tension the ADHD patient may experience. With this sort of anxiety, individuals may feel keyed up, continually worrying, and on edge. They may also experience the physical symptoms of anxiety such as an increase of sweating, fast heartbeat, cold and clammy hands, dry mouth, tingling feelings, upset stomach, hot or cold spells, frequent urination, and flushing. These are the symptoms of a disorder called Generalized Anxiety Disorder. It responds to different drugs than ADHD and, if present, may require different drug therapy.

Many ADHD patients have found that large doses of caffeine reduce the symptoms of ADHD, but at the expense of producing symptoms like those found in persistent anxiety. Stimulant drugs in a proper dosage are not only better than caffeine, but they do not produce these unwanted physical symptoms.

Also, as we discussed in Chapter 4, it is very probable that ADHD predisposes adolescents and adults to alcohol and drug abuse and dependence, and ADHD may also be increased among adult alcoholics and substance abusers. Other associations we and others have noticed clinically are heavy tobacco use, increased consumption of caffeinated drinks, and, as noted earlier, difficulties with academic and occupational functioning, and impairment in relationships.

HEREDITY AND ADHD SYMPTOMS

In addition to such symptoms, certain patterns of behavior within the family may suggest the diagnosis of ADHD in an adult. If John and Mary Doe have an ADHD child and Mary clearly does not have ADHD or a history of ADHD in her family, the odds increase that John is carrying the disorder and may also have some symptoms himself. Similarly, if an adult is having the above problems and has a parent or brothers or sisters with similar problems, he should consider the possibility that he may have ADHD. In years past, neither one's siblings nor one's parents would be formally diagnosed by a psychiatrist or psychologist as having ADHD. But since the symptoms of ADHD are so obvious, it is possible to make an educated guess about the diagnosis. If a relative is continually restless, distracted, disorganized, hot tempered, impulsive, moody, and has drunk or smoked too much, the chances that he has ADHD are fairly high.

PSYCHOLOGICAL PROBLEMS WITH ADHD

Our ADHD patients frequently have special psychological problems. Not surprisingly, these are often continuations of similar problems in childhood. Like the children, they tend to be underachievers at work and in the home. On the job they not only fail to obtain promotions but tend to be fired frequently because of their disorganization and hot temper. Their households are often chaotic.

Learning Disorders also often persist, and ADHD adults have more than their share of difficulties in reading, spelling, and arithmetic. Confusion of right and left may also continue, along with reversal in numbers and letters. Obviously, problems of this kind can easily interfere with performance in a variety of different jobs.

Relational and Child-Rearing Complications

The relationship between partners is often strained and "dysfunctional," and we suspect that relationships involving an ADHD partner break up more often than those that do not. Most of the origins of these difficulties can readily be seen in the patients' ADHD traits. Their impulsivity, their temper, their failure to listen to their partner, and sometimes a lack of interpersonal sensitivity disturb their interpersonal relationships. These relationships are further stressed if the continuing obstinacy, bossiness, and stubbornness seen in many ADHD children are present. Communication is difficult. The ADHD person does not attend to the other's conversation. He may tune out and drift off following his own train of thought. Not having listened, he may interrupt his spouse in response to his own thoughts. So the spouse has not been heard and is receiving a reply to a question not asked. Communication breaks down. Many ADHD couples have been treated for communication problems when the communication problems were one symptom of the underlying ADHD problems and not the sole cause of the current ones.

Unpredictable moodiness is difficult to live with. It is tiring to always be walking on eggs. It is likewise tiring to attempt to cheer up the unpredictably sad or try to get the overly enthusiastic partner to look at things realistically. The difficulty of living with a person with a hot temper is not hard to understand. However, the way the ADHD person handles his anger aggravates things. His anger is "a flash in the pan"; after expressing himself he feels fine in five to ten minutes. This is unlike his wife who may feel upset for the remainder of the day. Disorganization, not planning ahead, can drive the non-ADHD partner wild. If he is the household administrator, she may be repeatedly anxious and upset when bill collectors phone them—because he has forgotten to pay the bills—when credit card limits top out, and when bank accounts have vanished with impulsive buying. The familial disorganization, economic pressures, and job instability can combine to make the partner anxious, depressed, angry, and insecure. Impulsivity in family decisions—taking or terminating a vacation on the spur of the moment, buying something they had agreed not to, commitments made and commitments broken on a moment's notice—can further aggravate the problems. And the problems may be harder to resolve because the ADHD person is both bossy and stubborn. The spouse cannot expect subtle and accurate perception by the ADHD patient. Like the children with ADHD, many adults with ADHD are socially imperceptive and self-centered. The self-centeredness does not mean they like themselves. It simply means they have not learned how to place themselves in other people's shoes. This lack of awareness by the ADHD patient further torments his spouse because he has a serious difficulty in understanding, empathizing, and recognizing the nature and intensity of her feelings.

The ADHD parent is likely to have difficulty with his children. His personality may make it very difficult for him to parent children who have no problems. Unfortunately, he is very likely to be the parent of children with problems, ADHD problems. His inconsistency, lack of follow-through, unpredictability, and temper may produce behavioral problems even in a child who has no ADHD symptoms. Very frequently he does have an ADHD child, and the interaction between his children and himself may repeat the relationship between his parents and himself as a child. This interaction can lead to a vicious circle, and the increased friction is likely to make all the predictable problems of childhood and adolescence worse. The normal adolescent often experiences depression, often rebels, often experiments unwisely with sex and drugs. If that adolescent is reprimanded by an ADHD adult whose temper and unpredictability would place him at the low end of the parenting skills chart, severe problems are likely to arise out of ones that might have been temporary.

These patients tend to be dissatisfied with their lives in general. As a result of numerous unsatisfying experiences and defeats, they often have low self-esteem. As one patient who was a baseball fan observed, when your life is characterized by no hits, no runs, and plenty of errors, you do not have a terrific view of yourself.

At the expense of being repetitious, I wish to emphasize that psychiatrists do not agree on how many and which of the symptoms of the Utah Criteria must be present to reach a diagnosis of ADHD in adults. Further, many of the symptoms I have just enumerated are seen in a variety of other psychiatric disorders. Even if a person is hyperactive and inattentive and has several of the other problems listed, he or she may have another psychiatric disorder. As I have noted, symptoms very similar to these are seen in adults who have depressions that are considered biological in origin. Obviously, anyone who is hyperactive or inattentive and has at least two of the five further problems I listed does indeed have problems that suggest the advisability of psychiatric evaluation. He or she may not have adult ADHD but would probably benefit from appropriate treatment of some kind.

DIAGNOSIS OF ADULT ADHD

These, then, are the problems seen in ADHD adults. How do we diagnose a patient? First, we must determine what he was like in childhood. Every adult with ADHD had ADHD as a child. If the adult did not have the ADHD symptoms I have discussed, some other psychological problem is present. One of the difficulties in diagnosing adults is that they often do not remember what they were like as children. In our research, we have dealt with this problem in three ways: we have instructed prospective patients to talk with their parents about their own problems during childhood, or we have asked to talk to the parents ourselves; we have requested the parents of prospective patients to fill out a questionnaire describing the psychological characteristics and problems that the patients had when they were children; and we have requested that the patients fill out a questionnaire in which they rate their own behavior in childhood. These questionnaires are reproduced in the Appendix.

For both the diagnosis and the evaluation of treatment, it is extremely important to have the help of the spouse, significant other, or parent of the adult with possible ADHD. This is because in one respect ADHD adults may be exactly like ADHD children: they do not realize their symptoms and they do not fully realize the changes medication may produce. The parents of ADHD children recognize that their ADHD children either do not perceive or will not acknowledge their problem. The children may agree that they are not doing well in school or that they are having difficulty with peers, siblings, or their parents, but they rarely acknowledge responsibility for these problems (or the role that their behavior plays in causing these problems). The same imperceptiveness is often seen in ADHD adults. Partly it may be due to psychological self-protection. Not only do we not like to disclose our problems to other people, but we also do not like to disclose them to ourselves. Failure to perceive one's problems is a psychological protection method used not only by individuals with psychiatric difficulties of various kinds but by most of the rest of the world as well.

Another reason the ADHD adult may be blind to his psychological imperfections is that he has lived his whole life with them. In contrast, individuals who develop psychiatric disorders recognize the changes immediately: they will tell us how and when they began to feel depressed or became anxious or developed phobias. By comparison, the patient with ADHD has had the disorder his entire life. He is in some respects like someone with color blindness. The difference is that the person with color blindness learns about his disability as soon as he applies for a driver's license. He discovers that the two shades of gray that he sees are called "red" and "green" by most people. The ADHD patient may never realize that he has a disorder and, indeed, until very recently, most ADHD patients did not know there was an adult condition called ADHD. When he does discover that he has ADHD and learns what its symptoms are, he may for the first time look back on his life and see how the ADHD symptoms have been involved with his performance in school, his career, and his relationships with the important people in his life. As patients develop an understanding of what has happened, they typically experience two feelings. One is the awareness that this disorder has had major effects on who they became, who they are, and what they have done. The second may be a feeling of relief in finally understanding why things in their life have gone the way they have. However, realization is a two-edged sword and they may experience regret that they have suffered all their lives from a condition that could be treated and might have prevented their recurring and continuing difficulties.

Because of the difficulty of recognizing ADHD and distinguishing it from other disorders, it is important that someone with problems of this kind not attempt to diagnose himself. The previous descriptions are designed to serve as a list of warning symptoms that can alert the reader to the presence of problems that should be evaluated by a trained professional. A more complete discussion of the diagnostic tools used in the professional evaluation of patients suspected of having ADHD can be found in the Appendix.

DRUG TREATMENT OF THE
ADHD ADULT

■

As with the ADHD child, medication is the most effective treatment for adults with ADHD. When medication works, and it does so in about two-thirds of our patients, the effects are often dramatic. Many patients in our experimental programs had received treatment with both medication and psychotherapy before we had seen them. Because the symptoms of adult ADHD are similar in some respects to certain types of depressions, many patients had been given the standard medications employed in depression. In general, they had not been treated with the type of medications we have found most effective: stimulant drugs. Other drugs are also sometimes used, but these stimulants are the chief therapeutic agents.

STIMULANT DRUGS

As with children, stimulants are the most effective drugs. The stimulant drugs we have found most useful are the amphetamines (Dexedrine, Desoxyn, and Adderall), Ritalin, and Cylert. When effective, these drugs produce the following results.

Effectiveness

Inattentiveness and distractibility

Both these characteristics are reduced by stimulant medications. Responding patients find that they can focus their attention better on academic and office work, reading for pleasure, television, and movies. In addition, they are able to attend more to what people are saying and are more sensitive to mood and attitude changes in others. Because bad listening skills are a frequent cause of marital and family discord, being able to pay better attention to what others say and to what others want and don't want cannot help improving interpersonal relations. Increased attentiveness of this kind is not a paradoxical response. Anyone who takes stimulant medication in low doses may report that he concentrates better, and this may affect how he approaches necessary tasks. However, in contrast to the effect on the ADHD adult, it is not clear how useful this is for the normal person.

Hyperactivity

When present, fidgetiness, restlessness, and discomfort at being sedentary all disappear. Fingers and heels stop tapping, feet stop jiggling, and the treated patient will report that he can sit through a TV program or movie with much greater ease. At the same time, overall physical and mental energy is not decreased.

Impulsivity

The decrease in impulsivity can be observed in a small way on a day-to-day basis and also over a longer period of time. Patients successfully treated with stimulants think before they talk—they "engage their mind before they put their mouth in gear." They also converse more usefully. The ADHD child and adult frequently interrupt—they cannot wait to get their words in and further disrupt conversations. Impulsivity toward children changes: parents scream and hit less. Because sudden surges of feeling are less likely, the chances of strained or broken relationships also diminish. Impulse buying, spending sprees, and perhaps certain compulsive-impulsive activities, such as gambling, decrease.

To a greater extent, the patient considers the consequences of his behavior and acts accordingly.

Mood problems

When effective, medication removes both the highs and the lows. The normal person who takes amphetamines is likely to become euphoric—that is, he may develop an inappropriate intense feeling of pleasure (as in some mental illnesses). Such euphoria can lead to possible misuse and addiction. The ADHD patient, however, does not become euphoric: he is less bored, less discontented, and happier with his lot; in addition, his overexcitement goes away. If he has a clinical depression as well, depressed symptoms will persist. Clinical depression is not improved by stimulants.

Organization

Patients improve their planning. Students, homemakers, and wage earners begin to devote more thought to the organization of their daily activities. One sees such concrete results as homework and papers completed on time, improved regulation of children's activities, better meal preparation, better care of house and yard, prompt bill payment, and improved meeting of job deadlines. As a result, relations improve with both spouses and employers.

Hot temper

Effective treatment lengthens the patient's fuse and raises his boiling point—successfully treated patients explode less frequently and more mildly. The effects on a household may be profound. Since ADHD children tend to have ADHD parents, the common family situation is a tense one—a very difficult child and a short-tempered parent. The best management of ADHD children requires planning and coolness, and the

ADHD parent is poorly equipped to deal with an ADHD child. The temper control and organizational changes produced by stimulant medication can help greatly. Even though the hot temper of ADHD adults tends to be short-lived, no one enjoys having to live with a person who cannot control himself. Again, interpersonal relations improve.

Management of stress

Successfully treated ADHD adults report that their stress tolerance goes up—they are less easily "hassled" or discombobulated. The continuing stresses and strains of everyday life make them less anxious, less depressed, and less confused. This obviously plays a role in their demonstrable better organization. It is hard to follow a plan systematically when your motivation and mood change from moment to moment.

MEDICATION MANAGEMENT

Dosage

The dosages that have proved effective in ADHD adults are as follows. In most instances, the doses of Dexedrine and Desoxyn have been between 15 and 45 milligrams a day (uncommonly up to 60), of Ritalin between 30 and 90 milligrams a day (uncommonly, up to 120 milligrams), and of Cylert between 37.5 and 150 milligrams a day; in some instances, larger doses may be employed. Of the regular forms, not the long-acting formulations, a dose of Cylert is effective for the longest period of time, Dexedrine and Desoxyn act for an intermediate period, and Ritalin for the least time. In most patients Ritalin lasts about two and a half to three hours, and the daily dosing may be 10 to 15 milligrams every two and a half hours six times a day. For Dexedrine dosing is usually 5 to 15 milligrams every 3 to 4 hours, three to four times a day. Many ADHD patients receiving these drugs are scheduled to take Ritalin or Dexedrine only three times a day. This may be inadequate—particularly for Ritalin—and they go in and out of symptom control all day long and report—accurately—that the drug does not work right! They are essentially correct—the drug works, but they are going through medication-free periods several times a day. Ritalin, Dexedrine, Desoxyn, and Adderall tablets (not Dexedrine Spansules) must be taken with religious precision. If the useful effect of a medication is only two to two and a half hours, the patient may have to take six doses a day to achieve a good therapeutic effect. ADHD patients are exactly the wrong people to have to follow such a schedule! The solution is technical. We have patients purchase one of several watches (one is the Timex "Iron Man"; another is the Casio "Countdown"; there may be others). These can be programmed in the morning to go off after a fixed amount of time and then are reset each time they signal. *With watches, almost all ADHD patients take their medication correctly. Without such watches, **almost no patients succeed**.* Since repeated dosing is difficult for some patients, the treating physician may wish to substitute a longer-acting dosage form intended to last for eight to twelve hours (but unfortunately the long-acting forms tend to vary unpredictably in their length of action). Dexedrine Spansules are marketed in 5-, 10-, and 15-milligram sizes, permitting gradual adjustment of dose. Dexedrine Spansules may last four to eight hours and must sometimes be taken two or (very rarely) three times a day. Ritalin is manufactured in a long-acting formulation. It comes in only one dosage size so that the dose cannot be adjusted, lasts usually no more than four hours, and it may be less effective than a 20-milligram tablet. As mentioned earlier, a formulation of Ritalin lasting up to twelve hours may soon be available.

Overall, Ritalin, Dexedrine, and Desoxyn seem equally effective, but some patients clearly respond better to one rather than another. Cylert's usefulness may be limited to ADHD patients for whom one expects abuse problems if prescribed Ritalin, Dexedrine, Desoxyn, or Adderall. Even in such cases, its serious life-threatening hazards—as discussed in Chapter 5—may preclude its use.

As mentioned, Adderall is a newly introduced combination of amphetamines and their salts. It contains dextroamphetamine (as in Dexedrine) and leveoamphetamine, a variant of equal or lower potency. The claim is that Adderall only needs to be administered two times per day, but this is not certain (as opposed to two to three times for Dexedrine and once or twice a day for Dexedrine Spansules). Adderall is marketed in 5-, 10-, 20-, and 30-milligram tablets, and a physician is more likely to administer it because it is much more convenient for a patient who needs 15 milligrams to take one-half of a 30-milligram tablet of Adderall, rather than three 5-milligram tablets of Dexedrine or Desoxyn. Because price is always a consideration, it would be prudent, keeping the dose constant, to compare the effectiveness and price of Adderall, Dexedrine, Desoxyn, and dextroamphetamine (generic Dexedrine).

Side Effects

The most common side effects of the stimulant drugs are appetite loss and, if the medication is taken too late in the day, difficulty falling asleep. The appetite loss and the resulting weight loss are short-lived, and after several weeks the patient's appetite returns to normal. The sleep-preventing effects, however, do not disappear with time. A common problem is that the therapeutic effect of the medication wears off while the arousing effect remains. For example, a dose of Dexedrine taken at 4:00 P.M. might provide psychological benefits until 9:00 or 10:00 P.M. but will keep the individual up long past midnight. One alternative is to take the last dose earlier in the day, but that means the good effects may disappear in the late afternoon and early evening. Another alternative is to give a small dose of a sedative "major tranquilizer" an hour before bedtime. These sedative drugs appear to counteract the arousing effect of the stimulant drug without interfering with its beneficial action the next day. The "major tranquilizers" are not abusable and patients do not become tolerant of them. The one most frequently used is Mellaril (thioridazine). Its *long-term* use *may* be associated with undesirable side effects and should be discussed with the treating physician. Another nonabusable sedative is the antidepressant trazodone. With trazodone there is a very small risk (1 in 8,000 patients) that a man may develop a powerful erection called priapism that does not go away. It must be treated immediately because continuation of the erection can lead to permanent impotence.

Another (uncommon) side effect of stimulant drugs is an increase in pulse and blood pressure and for this reason a physician will check blood pressure before treatment and at intervals thereafter. A normal maximum systolic (the higher) blood pressure is 140; the maximum normal diastolic (the lower) blood pressure is 90. If stimulant medications are producing significant improvement but are also producing an increase in blood pressure above normal limits, the use of antihypertensive (blood-pressure lowering) drugs should be considered. It is obviously preferable to give a patient only one medication and not a second to control the side effects of the first, but when treatment is producing life-changing effects, a patient usually wants to continue the medication.

Special Problems

Two major problems exist with stimulant medication, one medical and the other legal. The medical problem is that the medication does not work before the patient takes it in the morning and wears off before he goes to sleep at night. If he is a very difficult person to live with (e.g., with an explosive temper), then even with drug treatment there are still likely to be several bad hours a day, early in the morning and late in the evening. The patients themselves obviously do not like this roller-coaster effect. It can sometimes be avoided by the use of monoamine oxidase inhibitors or bupropion (Wellbutrin), which I describe below.

The second major problem with the amphetamines (Dexedrine and Desoxyn) and Ritalin—and Cylert to a much lesser degree—is that they can be abused. The amphetamines—"speed"—and Ritalin can produce powerful feelings of excitation and euphoria when taken in large doses, particularly when injected into a vein or smoked. Because serious drug abuse problems developed in the late 1960s, the federal government developed policies regulating the prescription of drugs that can be abused or produce addiction. Drugs are placed in four categories, with the highest representing the most abusable medications. Amphetamines and Ritalin have been placed in the highest category, which includes morphine. As mentioned earlier, this classification means that they can be prescribed for only one month at a time (with no refills), that written prescriptions must be used rather than telephone orders, that prescriptions cannot be dated for future use, and that prescriptions must be filled within ten days of their having been written. In many states copies of the prescription must be filed in duplicate or triplicate.

This understandable regulation complicates the medical management of ADHD. The amphetamines have been used in the practice of medicine since the 1930s. Whether wisely prescribed or not, many individuals took the same doses for long periods of time, claimed to benefit from them, and did not increase the dose taken. Although amphetamines were occasionally abused, the epidemic of amphetamine abuse did not begin until the drug era of the 1960s. What happened was that the amphetamine abuser found that he had to escalate the dosage, smoke the drug, or inject it. Eventually, some amphetamine addicts took several hundred milligrams several times a day over a period of several days—doses ten times as great as those used therapeutically in the treatment of ADHD. Ritalin has been abused much less that the amphetamines, either because it is less desirable or less readily available. Cylert is insoluble in water and cannot be administered by vein, and drug users apparently do not like the effect it produces. The important scientific question here is whether the ADHD adult who might benefit from the comparatively low doses of Dexedrine, Desoxyn, and Ritalin that are useful therapeutically might obtain the highs associated with abuse if he took much larger doses or used the drugs intravenously. Unfortunately, we have no information with which to answer this question.

Because Dexedrine, Desoxyn, and Ritalin are known as highly abusable drugs, psychiatrists and other physicians are reluctant to use them in adults, particularly ADHD patients with problems of alcohol or substance abuse. That is one of the reasons our ADHD adults were treated with agents other than stimulants before they were referred to us. Thus, ironically, ADHD adults have been the least likely to be treated with the drugs that in our experience have been most effective—the stimulant drugs.

OTHER DRUGS

Other drugs that may be effective in adults with ADHD are the cyclic antidepressants and the antidepressants venlafaxine and bupropion. The use of antidepressants in children was discussed in Chapter 5.

Cyclic Antidepressants

The cyclic antidepressants have been used in the treatment of major (clinical) depression for forty years. They are not abusable. The initial response to the cyclic antidepressants may be in hours, rather than weeks (as in depression), but their effect is almost always considerably *less* than that of the stimulants. Patients often become tolerant to their effects, and the tolerance is not reversed by increasing their dose. Side effects include dry mouth, constipation, weight gain, lowered blood pressure when standing, decreased sexual interest, and impaired sexual functioning. The most commonly used are Tofranil (imipramine) and Norpramin (desipramine); doses are between 25 and 150 milligrams once a day.

Venlafaxine

A recently introduced antidepressant, Effexor (venlafaxine), is reported to be effective in ADHD adults, but it does not appear to be anywhere near as effective as the stimulants. It has a lesser effect on concentration problems and disorganization. It remains to be determined how many patients it helps, how much improvement occurs, and whether tolerance develops. It diminished sexual interest and large doses increase blood pressure in a small percentage of people.

Bupropion

Wellbutrin (bupropion) was developed in the 1980s as a drug to treat ADHD in children and is now marketed for the treatment of depression. As a treatment for ADHD in adults, it appears to work in a smaller percentage of patients than do the stimulants. As mentioned, larger experimental trials have been conducted and we hope to learn more about how effective it is in relieving ADHD symptoms and in what fraction of patients. It does not seem to control as many ADHD symptoms as the stimulants, and has less of an effect on improving concentration problems and organization. It apparently is not a long-acting drug. The dosage is usually prescribed as 150 to 300 milligrams, given in three divided doses. (It has recently been marketed in a "sustained release"

form in 100-milligram and 150-milligram tablets.) The usual
dose is 150-milligrams twice daily. The principal side effects
are irritability and insomnia.

JUDGING RESPONSE TO MEDICATION

Like children with ADHD, adults with ADHD do not recognize their problems initially and then may fail to notice
their progress after treatment. As indicated in the following
anecdotes, the judgment of another person is highly desirable
in measuring improvement.

Some months after our completion of a research study of
Cylert, I was stopped in the hall of the medical center by a
nurse I did not know. She introduced herself and said, "I'd
like to thank you very much." I replied: "You're welcome.
What did I do?" It turned out that her husband had participated in a drug study, and that the medication had had a
dramatically beneficial effect on their marriage. It had been
deteriorating over several years and, despite counseling, the
couple had been rapidly approaching divorce. The nurse stated that the stimulant medication had produced a pronounced
change in her husband's behavior, and with its help they had
been able to iron out their chronic problems. I had not treated
the patient and asked his treating physician about him. Although we generally query spouses or others in our drug studies, that had not been possible in this instance because the
nurse was away caring for her sick mother during the time
of the drug trial. The treating physician had rated the patient
as slightly improved—by the patient's judgment. By the
wife's judgment, however, a dramatically marked improvement took place.

The same phenomenon occurred in my treatment of another patient in a research study. Each week, I reviewed the
core symptoms of ADHD and asked the patient whether and
how much he had improved, worsened, or if he had stayed

the same. One week, when both the patient and his wife had come to see me, he answered my questions about restlessness, inattentiveness, organization, and temper by saying that each symptom was slightly improved. His overall judgment was also that he was "slightly improved." When he said this, his wife looked at him in surprise, placed her hand on his knee, looked me in the eye, and said, "Slightly improved! It's like being married to a different man!"

In both cases, the patient's inaccurate self-observation was the adult equivalent of the ADHD child's lack of awareness of his problems and of the change in behavior in response to medication.

WHEN AND HOW LONG TO TREAT WITH MEDICATION

The question of when to treat with medication arises because ADHD problems can be present in differing degrees, and both serious and milder symptoms may respond to treatment. The practical questions involve how much benefit is achieved with medication and what the risks are of its long-term use. Cost-benefit questions of this kind, of course, frequently occur in other areas of life as well as in medicine. To the best of our current knowledge, the risks incurred by long-term treatment with stimulant medication are very low. In the era before restrictions were placed on the use of stimulant medications, tens of millions of people took them without addiction, and no epidemic of serious medical problems was reported. So far as allergies and unusual reactions are concerned, the amphetamines and Ritalin appear to be much safer than aspirin or penicillin. Allergic reactions are so uncommon that doctors who treat children with these medications have abandoned periodic blood testing to detect allergy. Still, the medications do increase heart rate, and in some individuals they raise blood pressure slightly. There are no other known long-term effects. And to balance this potential side effect, it is important to recognize the health-promoting effects that stimulant drugs have in some ADHD people. Some patients find that stimulants reduce their need for nicotine, making it easier for them to give up smoking. Some adults with ADHD have given up excessive drinking. Others have, with the help of medication, organized their lives and enjoyed a less stressful existence. Such health-promoting effects must be weighed against the blood pressure effects already noted. Furthermore, if blood pressure is raised to an *excessive level* yet stimulant treatment is clearly beneficial, the physician can add another medication to lower blood pressure.

From a practical standpoint, clinicians who treat patients with ADHD find that they tend to request treatment when their lives have become difficult, take medicine and with its help straighten out their lives, and then often discontinue medication until the next emergency arises. This may not be the wisest policy for an ADHD adult to follow because he is frequently unaware of the effects of his disorder on others; when he discontinues medication he may be destroying personal relationships, producing family turmoil, and impairing job success without awareness. Periodic use of medication is a good idea if the patient and his significant other learn to recognize when his supposedly mild ADHD is causing problems that he does not usually perceive. The basic policy for the ADHD patient should be to make sure his problems are not hurting himself or others. To make this assessment, he generally needs the help of a partner.

PSYCHOLOGICAL THERAPIES
FOR THE ADHD ADULT

■

An essential component in the psychological treatment of the ADHD adult is education. The patient must learn to recognize which symptoms of ADHD cause the most difficulties in everyday life. Such self-awareness does not come easily. Most of us do not know how we appear to others—we are all surprised to hear our voice on audiotape or see ourselves on videotape—but it is probably more important for the ADHD patient to see himself clearly. The Scottish poet Robert Burns observed in a famous poem, "O wad some Pow'r the giftie gie us / To see oursels as others see us!" and continued in less well-known lines, "It wad frae monie a blunder free us / An' foolish notion." The powers may have given us the opposite kind of gift: not to see ourselves as others see us. Many of us can get by without such self-observation, but the ADHD adult cannot.

How education of the ADHD adult is best accomplished and what kinds of psychological therapy are best are not certain. Couple therapy, group therapy, support groups, and psychological counseling from a clinician familiar with ADHD may all have their usefulness.

Most of our patients have had spouses or other partners, so the approach we use is derived from standard techniques of couple therapy. Each partner examines the behavior of the other, focusing especially on three aspects of the relationship: communication, expectations, and stylized patterns of behavior.

Frequently, marital partners have never learned to talk to each other—to say what they think, feel, and want. They hope that somehow their mates can read their minds. When this doesn't happen, they feel frustrated and become angry. Consequently, persuading marriage partners to say what is on their minds has been found therapeutically useful. Often just this step can result in some modification of behavior. Partners can also improve communication by making sure that, when they do express themselves, the other person has understood the message correctly—has the facts straight and understands the intention.

With better communication, the partners are less likely to act in terms of unrealistic expectations derived from previous experiences in their own families or even from an over-romantic popular culture. Each member of a couple has to learn what the partner's actual desires and capabilities are, and sometimes this may mean modification of original rosy dreams about gourmet meals every day, athletic sexual performance on demand, and immaculate, well-behaved children.

In approaching established behavior patterns that may produce marital conflict, therapists help the partners explore such questions as who sets the household rules, whose friends are seen, who does what chores, who spends more time with the children, who decides how money is spent, and who initiates sexual activity. In examining important elements of their life together, the partners begin to recognize particular behaviors (from squeezing the toothpaste tube in the middle to over-drawing bank accounts) that have become sources of trouble. When the various irritants are brought into the open, the couple becomes aware of the need to compromise. Sometimes the therapist can help them by suggesting specific behavioral techniques, such as "bargaining contracts" or a "reward system," which can achieve a better division of household responsibilities.

When one member in a couple has ADHD, the kinds of problems that usually emerge in couple therapy are likely to be greater because of such factors as impulsivity and hot temper. The therapist's focus on better communication not only helps the couple to deal with the problems of living together but is an important part of the process whereby the ADHD adult learns to identify individual difficulties.

Whether other techniques would be helpful needs to be determined. In particular, it might be very useful to treat ADHD adults in groups. The group setting would provide the opportunity for them to observe their own and other ADHD patients' behavior in the here and now—they and others can see the behavior as it happens. Group therapy can offer a variety of benefits: support and reassurance as the patients discover that their problems are not unique; an opportunity to express feelings that may be repressed at home or on the job; frank assessments of interpersonal behavior; a testing ground for experimenting with other ways of behaving; recognition and praise from others when behavioral improvement occurs; a situation in which the patient can be of help to others. In addition, when groups are composed of patients who are at various levels of sophistication (from the novice to the patient who has already learned a great deal about his problems), valuable education can occur among the patients themselves.

Group techniques have been useful in teaching patients with various psychiatric disorders about their problems, the manifestation of these problems in everyday life, and their treatment. It is therefore very likely that group therapy would be helpful to ADHD adults, but careful research is needed to demonstrate its usefulness.

Psychological self-healing or self-development might be another avenue worth exploring. With the help of medication an ADHD adult is more in control and presumably has an increased ability to change himself. The behaviors to monitor would be those that had created difficulties for him in the past: temper, impulsivity, disorganization, alcohol or substance abuse. Related psychological support groups for certain behaviors might be considered, such as Alcoholics Anonymous or Narcotics Anonymous. To help with real-world problems caused by past behaviors, such measures as debt consolidation or vocational retraining could even be considered. By whatever means the ADHD adult seeks to change his life, the point is that medical treatment allows a kind of psychological stability to occur so that such patients can learn *by themselves* new techniques of avoiding or solving problems and correcting their own deficiencies.

Not all problems can be helped with the approaches of couple therapy, group therapy, or self-development. Some patients might benefit from a "general insight" offered by a clinician knowledgeable about ADHD. As has been made clear earlier, the ADHD adult has usually been chronically unsuccessful. He quite likely had a difficult, even unhappy childhood and adolescence. He has low self-esteem, a history of academic and vocational underachievement, and troubled personal relationships. For some ADHD patients, psychological treatment that focuses on the consequences of the main symptoms of ADHD might be of great benefit. A clinician familiar with treating ADHD can explain what has happened to the patient: why relationships with parents, siblings, and teachers were difficult in the past; why relationships with partner, children, and coworkers may be difficult now; why the patient feels he has not been successful in any endeavor ever attempted; and what behaviors bring on unwanted consequences. Even if the patient is taking medication for ADHD, certain patterns of behavior may persist.

Finally, it must be remembered that in addition to special difficulties associated with their disorder, ADHD adults may have the kinds of other problems that anyone is likely to have. When ADHD symptoms are controlled, some patients find themselves faced with problems that had remained hidden and that they now must tackle. However, a majority are pleased with the progress they have made and are content to face life's challenges with their newfound awareness of their specific problems and with their newfound help—medication.

TREATMENT OF MILDER ADHD DISORDERS AND OF ADHD IN COMBINATION WITH OTHER DIAGNOSES

■

The Utah Criteria—the ones provided in this chapter—were constructed to be very specific because the research we were doing was controversial. We wanted to make our requirements so tight that individuals meeting them were most likely to have ADHD. We knew that by doing this we would fail to study individuals who did not meet the full diagnostic rules for the diagnosis of ADHD. When one talks to the parents, brothers, and sisters of ADHD individuals, one is impressed with the apparently increased number of ADHD symptoms these individuals have that are not sufficient to label them as full-fledged ADHD. This is not unexpected since in most all disorders one finds varying degrees of severity of the same illness. Talking to the relatives of ADHD adults we find people with varying combinations—for example, of chronic inattentiveness, unstable mood, disorganization, or explosive temper. No one has investigated whether these mild, possible forms of ADHD would respond to the same treatment that is effective in treating full-fledged ADHD. Physicians have been reluctant to treat these minor forms for three reasons. First, full-fledged ADHD has been a controversial diagnosis. Second, psychiatrists are reluctant to use potentially abusable drugs in patients who are less certain to have ADHD and in whom abuse would presumably be more likely to occur. Third, psychiatrists have been cautious about treating minor symptoms of ADHD—for example, chronic inattentiveness—with stimulant medication because those symptoms may be manifestations of another psychiatric disorder. Many people with anxiety, depression, and other clinical psychiatric disorders have serious problems with attention and treating them with stimulants would be incorrect treatment.

Although the strict guidelines of our research studies mandated that we exclude patients with clinical depression, in my clinical practice I have treated patients who reported symptoms of both ADHD and major depression. I found that these patients generally benefited from treatment with a stimulant drug plus an antidepressant. An antidepressant by itself may control the symptoms of depression but not affect the ADHD symptoms. Similarly, a stimulant drug may benefit the ADHD symptoms but not the depression. Appropriate treatment requires the use of both types of medication. I have had several patients who appeared to develop such a depression in the course of extended treatment for their ADHD. One was a forty-year-old woman with prominent ADHD symptoms as well as a disturbed sleep pattern of multiple anxious awakenings throughout the night. She did not have symptoms of clinical depression: she was interested in things, experienced no guilt, and felt that life was worth living. On Ritalin both her ADHD symptoms and her abnormal sleep problems resolved. A year and a half later, while doing well on stimulants, she began to develop symptoms of biological depression with loss of interest in pleasure in almost all her activities. Ritalin was continued but Paxil, an antidepressant, was administered. Within eight weeks her interest in life resumed. She remained on the Ritalin and the antidepressant was diminished after nine months with no reappearance of her symptoms. She is being followed carefully, because once an individual has had one clinical depression, he or she is more likely to have a recurrence.

I will discuss briefly another case to illustrate the presence of ADHD with another diagnosis. A thirty-five-year-old woman came to me after having been in and out of multiple psychotherapies for twelve years and psychiatric treatment for three years. Her initial problem had been recurring depressions that appeared to have developed in reaction to continuing difficulties in her life. The psychotherapist had interpreted the depression as a response to a bad marriage and two difficult children. However, her depression continued after she divorced and remarried, this time happily. After twelve years of unsuccessful treatment, her therapist referred her to a psychiatrist interested in clinical depression. She was placed on tricyclic antidepressants (the older antidepressant that are, however, just as effective as the newer drugs for depression), and most of her depressive symptoms resolved.

When questioned about her childhood she mentioned that in addition to family problems she had been a tomboy, not much of a student, and "tough," stubborn, and bossy. Regarding her temperament at present, the physician discovered that she could not concentrate on reading or organize the running of the household; she was very distractible, a never-ceasing bundle of energy, short tempered, and, as in childhood, stubborn and bossy. These were all temperamental features of her personality that may have contributed to the previous difficulties in her first marriage and developing problems in her second one. She was placed on Dexedrine and obtained considerable benefit, becoming more attentive, less driven, cooler tempered, better organized, less stubborn, and less bossy. Her second marriage improved considerably.

These last two cases illustrate that other psychiatric conditions can occur together with ADHD. ADHD does not increase the likelihood of a person developing them but it does not prevent one from developing them. Their presence will not likely be recognized by the nonpsychiatric physician—or by the nonpsychiatric nonphysician—with the result that their diagnosis is likely to be missed and the disorders therefore left untreated.

ILLUSTRATIVE CASE HISTORIES— ADHD ADULTS

■

In order to give the reader a "feel" for the disordered adults, I will present two sets of case histories. The first group consists of brief descriptions of the patients and their symptoms, the common themes in their childhoods, and the treatment deemed appropriate for each. The second group includes autobiographical accounts that dramatically demonstrate the powerful life-changing effects that treatment of ADHD in adults can have.

Patient Name: *Alan A*
Diagnosis: ADHD

Alan was a forty-seven-year-old man who came to a psychiatrist with complaints of increasing confusion, disorganization, and depression. He dated the onset of his problems to changes that had taken place in the real estate office in which he worked. He was second in command to his father who had recently suffered a stroke and was forced to retire. This was followed shortly by the retirement of the office manager, a woman who had run the office for thirty-five years with excessive control and attention to detail. Work had ceased going smoothly. In addition, the patient was no longer able to organize his life at home and the household was becoming increasingly disrupted. His wife, whom he described as a "marine sergeant," tried to fill all the gaps but was becoming exhausted. He had received multiple antidepressants and had sustained no substantial benefit.

Patient Name: *Barbara B*
Diagnosis: ADHD; history of Conduct Disorder traits

Barbara was a thirty-two-year-old mother of two ADHD boys who were being treated in a clinic. They had received medication that had improved their behavior considerably at school, but she still had great difficulty managing them at home. She was unable to provide any organization, schedules, or definite expectations. She overreacted to trivial provocations; lost her temper; and then set punishments that she never carried out (e.g., she would threaten to "ground" the boys for two weeks and one hour later forget that she had done so). She was seeing a psychologist who was attempting to teach her the principles of behavior management but without success. Her own life had been chronically disorganized. She had three children by three men, the first at age sixteen, and had never functioned successfully. She did poorly in high school and dropped out, occupied a number of brief menial jobs, and was receiving welfare. Her inability to organize her life, run her household, or take care of her children had required multiple therapy, by a variety of therapists, over many years.

Patient Name: **Carol C**
Diagnosis: ADHD, Inattentive Type, mild;
                Learning Disorders

Carol was a forty-two-year-old woman who had returned to work after her children left home. She obtained a job as a clerk in an office and functioned very well personally and very poorly occupationally. She had difficulty with word processing, wrote disorganized messages, and manifested spelling problems. She had some difficulty with alphabetization and filing. She confused appointments and forgot and mixed messages. Nonetheless, she was warm, friendly, well intentioned, and well liked.

Patient Name: **David D**
Diagnosis: ADHD, Hyperactive-Impulsive Type

David was a thirty-five-year-old man who appeared with his wife for treatment of chronic marital problems that had stemmed from David's personality. He was described by his wife as "loving and caring" but "impossible" to live with. He was responsible for the administrative running of the household but did an abysmal job. Bills were not paid on time and repairs were not made. Tax records were always misplaced and tax-payment time was a disaster. He would respond to the difficulties he had produced with brief outbursts of anger during which he would explode verbally, but not physically, and after *which he would quickly calm down. His good mood was restored in a matter of minutes, but his wife continued to be upset for the rest of the day. She found him difficult to be around because he was so restless. He did not sit still at the dinner table or in front of the TV and perennially tapped his foot and fingers. Impulsivity was also a problem: He spoke without thinking, hurting her feelings, upsetting the children, and antagonizing friends. He also had recurrent impulse buying that, although not for expensive items, added to the family debt. The couple received counseling and was given communication therapy without much benefit.*

COMMON THEMES IN THE LIVES OF ADHD ADULTS

The childhoods of these people carry several common themes.

Alan A had been a dreamy, distractible, absentminded, good-natured boy who never completed anything at home or at school. He would begin to clean his room and stop halfway. Homework assignments were never finished. Teachers complained of his dreaminess and absentmindedness. When he was interested in a subject—as he became in some fantasy games—he studied it intensely and often became very proficient. He was an underachiever at high school and college and graduated from college with a C average.

Barbara B had been a typical ADHD child with inattentiveness, hyperactivity, and impulsivity. She had a low normal intelligence. Although obedient until puberty, she then began to tear loose, staying away from home at night, going out with older men, and experimenting with alcohol and drugs. She left home at the age of sixteen to live with a nineteen-year-old ne'er-do-well who was alcoholic, infrequently employed, and who beat her. She stayed with him for two years and then left to raise their first child. This unfortunate choice of partners was repeated on two more occasions with similar results. The symptoms she showed in the psychologist's office were all continuations of those that she had had in childhood. She was noticeably and uninterruptedly restless, inattentive and distractible, impulsive in speech and behavior, disorganized, overreactive, and given to temper outbursts.

Carol C had been a pleasant underachieving child. She was somewhat inattentive and distractible, but obedient, well behaved and "sweet." She had marked difficulty learning to read and spell and had been placed in a resource room during elementary school. She never mastered reading or spelling and dropped out of high school in the tenth grade.

David D had been a rambunctious toddler and adolescent. Although somewhat inattentive, his major problems were his impulsivity and hyperactivity. His mood was unstable, he fought frequently, and was often involved in difficulty with teachers at school and with the principal. Nonetheless, he was well liked by his peers because he was gregarious and a good athlete. During late adolescence he went through a period of alcohol and marijuana abuse and dropped out of high school. He stopped his substance abuse on his own and obtained a GED at the age of twenty-one.

TREATMENT OF CASE SUBJECTS

Alan had symptoms of both ADHD and a biological depression. He was begun on a trial of Dexedrine and had marked change in a variety of behaviors. His concentration improved substantially, he became less distractible and better organized, and, with help from a new and effective secretary, was able to organize his work at the office. His functioning at home improved to a degree previously never shown. He started to organize and carry out his household duties appropriately, and became less dependent on his wife. Despite this improvement, he continued to have symptoms of depression with a loss of interest and pleasure. He was again given a trial of an antidepressant and after a period of several weeks his depressive symptoms diminished substantially. He was able to function at home and at the office, his self-esteem greatly increased, and for the first time in his life he became effective with his performance at work and home. The antidepressant was tapered and discontinued after a period of six months with no recurrence of the depression. The Dexedrine was maintained and the ADHD symptoms remained under control.

Barbara's clear-cut and persistent ADHD symptoms had not responded to counseling and, when seen by the psychiatrist, she was given a trial of Ritalin. This produced benefit in a number of areas. Her concentration and distractibility decreased and her explosive temper nearly disappeared. Because she was now attentive, she was able, with the aid of a therapist, to begin to plan and organize her life. Behavioral regimens were established for the children, and she was able to plan and execute them successfully. She continued to need and receive supportive therapy as well as medication. Her improved functioning led to plans for her to obtain a GED with the eventual hope of obtaining specific job training.

Carol had been slightly ADHD as a child, Inattentive Type, with clear-cut Learning Disorders. She had never mastered the skills necessary for clerical work. A trial of medication improved her attention slightly, but produced no improvement in her reading, spelling, and clerical ability. Because of her winning personality, the firm decided to keep her and positioned her as the receptionist. She functioned extremely well in this role. She continued to be well liked by her employer and by customers and performed satisfactorily.

David had been an ADHD child, primarily hyperactive and impulsive type. He was given a trial of Ritalin and had a dramatic response. The least important but most immediate effect was that his hyperactivity disappeared. He stopped tapping his foot all day long. His temper cooled considerably. Whatever happened physiologically, he described himself as being able to "count to ten" and rarely exploded. He became more patient and was able to plan and organize activities around the home. His impulsivity also decreased. He reported that he found himself listening to what other people were saying, and, rather than "just put in my two cents," learning to contain himself and follow the conversation. His impulsive buying decreased substantially and over time virtually disappeared.

The following case histories illustrate the kinds of changes that can occur when medication reduces symptoms and adult ADHD patients have the opportunity to experience psychological growth. When medicine works, it does so quickly. Symptoms such as hyperactivity and concentration problems may be alleviated almost immediately. Psychological growth, however, occurs much more slowly. Patients with ADHD have a lifelong history of psychological maladjustment. An immediate improvement in their concentration does not immediately better their interpersonal relationships, their vocational activities, or their approach to life. But the medication, when effective, allows time for psychological change to occur and, though the rate of change may be gradual, the cumulative effect can be profound.

These accounts by patients and their spouses are taken from my book *Attention-Deficit Hyperactivity Disorder in Adults* (Oxford University Press, New York, 1995).

THE EXPERIENCES OF ADHD ADULT PATIENTS ON STIMULANTS

The following accounts by four patients (Daniel P, Caroline G, Sonia D, and George F) and two spouses (writing about George F and Bruce C) communicate a sense of the relief some adult ADHD patients and their families experience when treatment with Ritalin (methylphenidate) begins. The history by Sonia D conveys an idea of changes experienced on both amphetamine and Ritalin. All the accounts also vividly describe what it is like to be afflicted with ADHD.

DANIEL P

■

COMMENT BY DR. WENDER

Daniel P, a thirty-one-year-old married father of two, referred himself to the clinic with complaints that "More and more I am aware that I am different from other people—I can't get things done—I have no stick-to-itiveness." He stated that he rarely lasted in any job for more than six months. He was not fired—he got bored and would leave. His easy susceptibility to boredom penalized him at college, which he had begun on several occasions, never lasting more than a few months.

He states that he had had chronic difficulties in associating with other people. He has never had a close friend or a confidant. In company he has always found himself doing things inappropriately and has been embarrassed by his own behavior. When invited by other people, he feels they don't like him. He also feels that he cannot participate in the conversational trivia that often happens in group meetings.

Boredom has been a chronic problem. He will watch a movie and read at the same time. While watching television he continually flips the channels. He has had chronic difficulty with anger. As a child he stole powder from his father's shotgun shells and used it to fire cannons. He chased his sisters with knives until the age of fifteen or sixteen: "I thrived on making them cry." The other things he would do to upset them was to put his fingers in their food and twist their arms. He learned to turn some anger inward as a child and prevented his expressing it more fully by resorting to imaginative, gory science-fiction-like inventions. As an adult, when angry, he had put his fist through the wall. His marriage has lasted because his wife was very calm and obliging.

His course in the study had been as follows: in the placebo-controlled trial he showed a moderate to marked response to Ritalin and has continued in the study for the past eight years on a dose of 50 milligrams a day (10 milligrams every three hours, five times per day). On medication his temper has been controlled, he is not bored, he has shown little insta-bility of mood, and he has become extremely well organized. As a consequence, his relationship with his wife improved substantially, and he was able to obtain the position of a re-ligious teacher and has been able to function very well in that role. His score on the scale of psychological and occu-pational functioning improved from "moderate to serious symptoms (anxiety and depression) or moderate to severe im-pairment in social or occupational functioning" to "if symp-toms are present, they are short-lived and expectable re-sponses to psychological or social pressures with no more than slight impairment in social or occupational function-ing," and his score on the scale of social adjustment has improved from "moderate maladjustment" to "excellent ad-justment."

STATEMENT BY DANIEL P

It is difficult to know where to begin. My goal is to explain what it is like to have Attention-Deficit Hyperactivity Dis-order as an adult. But I believe it is impossible for "normal" people to understand the frustration, anger, confusion, and eventual hopelessness that comes with failure at every turn. I will do my best, but please understand, I am attempting to tell apples and oranges what it feels like to be a banana.

I am an adult male of thirty-one years. About eight years

ago I met Dr. Paul H. Wender for the first time. The meeting was painful. Whether he intended it or not, I don't know, but his questions became increasingly irritating. Not for content, but because of the seemingly unimportant gibberish. I have come to realize that those questions were important, but the experience illustrates the frustration that comes with the inability to focus or understand. This was a very common experience throughout my life.

Inevitably, this frustration leads to fits of acting out and even violence. While these results seem related, the causes are different. The acting out comes from a need to do something. The something could be anything that crossed my mind. On one occasion in high school my science teacher had assigned us several pages of textbook busy-work. Everyone was working so hard and the class was so silent, but the work was so senseless that I stood on my desk, screamed at the top of my lungs and ran across the tops of the desks, then returned to my desk and continued the assignment. The teacher was either too shocked, too amused (along with the class), or too stupid to do anything about it. I, on the other hand, was mortified at my actions. When I said there was a "need to do something," that need is genuine—so overpowering that it forced me to do things I normally would not. There is no rhyme or reason, it simply had to be done.

The other result of frustration—violence—was actually the release of anger that I felt at all times. Always just below the surface, I had a seething volcano of anger and violence ready to explode. I played football in Little League and again in high school, and I enjoyed hitting and hurting others. There was such a tremendous sense of relief to hit and to hurt. When someone would limp off or have to be carried off the field, the feeling was near ecstasy. Even now as I write this I can remember those feelings. I don't understand them, but I remember them.

The anger also caused me to constantly look for a release. I wanted someone to provoke me so I could hurt them. This anger could not be eaten up by physical exercise or other releases. It typically was just there, and I was forced to deal with it. My parents, who were very strict, forced me to learn control. Which I did, but the anger was always there, waiting.

Another effect that I can now recognize was an inability to read and study. On countless occasions I would attempt to study for school and fail miserably. After only a few minutes I would become so irritated that I would throw the book across the room and watch television instead. The biggest problem was my inability to stay focused. I could read pages in a text while my mind was elsewhere, settling an old argument I had had with a friend two years ago, or beaming aboard the Star Ship Enterprise. I could read the words, I just couldn't attach any meaning.

Much of this led to the last effect that I am aware of, and that is guilt. I have felt guilt for everything I have ever done and many things I didn't do. Please do not suppose me guilty of any great wrongdoing, but things like hitting one of my sisters, lying to my mom, saying the wrong thing at a party, or simply being the life of the party. Afterwards, even after admitting my lies or apologizing, I was still racked with guilt. Similarly, in situations when I should have done something and didn't, the guilt was also very real. Like remembering when I meant to tell a foul-mouthed man on the bus to shut his yap, but didn't, can be a particular source of pain. My mind would return me to the instance time and time again. I would imagine that I acted properly each time, but it never helped. Some of these moments are decades old. There was an incident where I embarrassed myself on stage when I was in elementary school in front of the entire student body that had bothered me until I met Dr. Wender.

Hopefully, I have given some kind of an understanding of my experience. Although most illustrations were from my younger years, rest assured they continued well into adulthood. In fact, things had gotten so bad that I was becoming a recluse and refused to mingle with other people. It was then

I realized I needed help and was eventually introduced to Dr. Wender. As I said, his first interview was almost more than I could stand, but after being placed on 10 milligrams of Ritalin five times daily, I have sincerely enjoyed our meetings and even looked forward to them. My wife told Dr. Wender that the change had been dramatic. I was a little slower to recognize the change. Frustration was only a memory, the "need" as well as the seething anger were gone, and for the first time I opened a college textbook and read it from cover to cover with good understanding. Not just reading it, mind you, but outlining and taking notes. The experience frightened me because I was actually understanding nearly all of it. That gave me the courage to return to college full-time and finish my degree, which I have done. I can think clearly, I can discuss without getting frustrated, I can argue without losing control, and most wonderful of all, I can read! I have discovered the wonderful world of literature. But that's not all; for the first time since my first job when I was fourteen, I have kept a job longer than six months and actually have a professional career.

There is one more thing, for lack of a better word, that Ritalin has changed. There were times that my mind would seem to engage without my knowledge or consent. And I would be stranded on a runaway locomotive that would crash through any barrier I would erect in attempts to gain control. This would happen most often as I lay in bed waiting for sleep. The mental locomotive might take a trip that lasted all night. Sometimes it might engage in the middle of the night and wake me from a dead sleep. Ritalin stopped this. On more than one occasion I have asked Dr. Wender to convince me that Ritalin is a stimulant because on those nights of the thought express, I take Ritalin and it's like the calm after an ocean storm. The waves are slowly subdued until the surface is like shimmering glass and sleep comes so naturally that I enter REM easily. Sometimes I will wake up exactly two and a half hours after taking the first dose and need to take a second. Again the storm passes and sleep returns. On rare occasions I might awake having not taken any Ritalin before bed, but a dose then has the same calming effects.

There is no way to explain what Dr. Wender and his treatment of me with Ritalin means to me. Ritalin is a true miracle drug. It saved my education, my marriage, and quite possibly my life. Ritalin has given me what I thought was impossible, control of my life. And although I'm still a banana, at least I'm a little more spherical and can roll with the punches.

CAROLINE G

■

COMMENT BY DR. WENDER

Caroline G, a thirty-two-year-old mother of two boys, contacted our clinic after reading an article given her by one of her son's teachers. She had enrolled in a community college computer program, but homework was a terrible problem because she could not stick with it. Caroline experienced chronic distractibility, impulsivity, an explosive temper, and an inability to sustain long-term relationships. During the entire initial evaluation she was swinging on her chair.

Caroline met the criteria for a diagnosis of Attention-Deficit Hyperactivity Disorder and was entered into a trial of Ritalin and placebo. She showed a moderate to marked improvement on Ritalin and was then entered into the long-term phase of the study. After one year in the study she reported that she had quit smoking and drinking on her own. She has continued for nine years on a dose of 50 milligrams of Ritalin per day (10 milligrams every two and a half hours, five times per day). Her score on a scale of overall psychological occupational functioning improved from moderate to slight symptoms and moderate to slight impairment in social and occupational functioning. Her score on the scale of social adjustment improved from "moderate-to-severe maladjustment" to "excellent adjustment."

STATEMENT BY CAROLINE G

I've been asked to write this letter to describe how Ritalin has helped and changed my life. Before I can describe the changes, I feel it necessary to give a little background on myself so that you can better understand how I have benefited from the use of Ritalin over the years.

I grew up in a very dysfunctional home as a child. Although my family, specifically my parents, tried to keep up the appearance of normality, it was anything but a normal childhood. My father was an alcoholic. Although I can never remember him staggering drunk, he was always drinking. As a loving parent, he was totally lacking. He never really involved himself in raising us, except when he had to, as in physically disciplining us.

My mother, on the other hand, did everything that was expected of a middle-class housewife—the PTA, Girl Scout Leader, Cub Scout Leader, etc. . . . although her heart wasn't really in it. She admitted to me several years ago that she hated it; she only did it because it was expected of her to keep up appearances. She portrayed the perfect loving mother to the world, while at home she showed us very little affection or love. I'm not even sure if my mother really loved any of her children, or even wanted us, and I think that even as a child I sensed this.

While I was growing up, my mother described me as her free spirit. I was always happy and on the go. Always getting into trouble, I did things on impulse without regard to the consequences of my actions. Most of the time I believed I wouldn't get caught, and, if caught, I would lie about it. I thought if I kept up the lie, they would eventually have to believe me. I was like a whirling dervish, always on the go, I couldn't sit still for any length of time, and if I had to stay in one place, I always had a body part moving, such as shaking my leg or fiddling with my hair.

As a child, I was very emotional, to the point of being overly dramatic. I would laugh too loud, cry constantly over little things, stupid things, my voice could carry over any conversation, and I was extremely aggressive with a very violent temper. My emotions ruled my life, making it difficult to fit in very well with my peers. I constantly would say inappropriate things to try to fit in, but I was basically a loner.

I didn't really do well in school for the first three years, although I was above average intelligence and could read before I entered kindergarten. I nearly failed in second grade. I can remember being frustrated with how slow the other children were. I would finish the lesson the teacher and class were doing and go on to the next lesson. Then when called on by the teacher to read or do a problem, I wouldn't be able to because I didn't know where we were. This caused the teacher to become very frustrated with me because my test scores were always very high but I couldn't keep my attention on what the class was doing. In the fourth grade I was lucky enough to get a teacher who recognized my problem and my potential and put me into an individual study program. At this time I started to get straight As. By the time I was in sixth grade, I was doing eighth-grade-level work. I managed to keep my grades up and graduate, although if I had been an average student, I probably would never have made it out of high school.

These problems followed me into my teen and adult years. Although I did extremely well in school, I still had trouble socializing with my peers. I was an overactive, talkative teenager; I was impulsive and I blurted out inappropriate things at the wrong time. Basically, I irritated other people. When I was fourteen years old, I started to drink alcohol, and when I was fifteen, I sought out the local drugs on the street. I started smoking marijuana first, then progressed by the time I was seventeen to painkillers (Percodan, Demerol), LSD, and cocaine. It wasn't until I started using drugs and alcohol that I was able to actually socialize with other teenagers. Not just those who partied, but also the kids who didn't. The use of marijuana slowed me down enough to stop and think before I acted. I became more comfortable in situations that used to be very stressful and difficult for me.

As an adult, I had problems with any kind of relationship. I could be friends with men, but on a dating-relationship level, I could never stay in one more than three or four months. I was still impulsive, spending money earmarked for bills. I had a serious drug and alcohol problem, and my self-esteem was in the basement.

After I had children, I found that I had another serious problem. I had no patience and no control over my temper. I became fearful of hurting my own children. I took parenting courses, and had several classes in child and adolescent psychology in college, but even with all these courses, it didn't help when disciplining my children. There were times when I actually felt like beating my kids senseless. I couldn't understand how I could feel this way when I loved my children. It got to the point where any little thing would make me break into tears. Sometimes, I would cry for no reason. I knew I wasn't depressed because I was always happy. But my mood swings were driving me crazy. One minute I would be mad, the next a raging maniac, then I would start crying, and then I would be fine as if nothing had happened—all in the span of five or six hours. I would get depressed, but it would never last more than a day or two. Sometimes I felt as if I was going crazy.

Since I have been involved in the Ritalin study at the University of Utah Medical Center, my whole life has changed for the better. I finally feel normal. My mood swings are almost gone. They could almost be considered normal. I don't explode or blow up over little things anymore. I have more patience with my children and have been able to institute a more consistent form of discipline without the physical violence that permeated my discipline before.

I have better control over my impulsivity. My financial situation has improved considerably and I no longer find myself spending money recklessly. I have even stopped my drinking and use of drugs without having to go through any kind of counseling or rehabilitation. I find that I just don't have the desire to do them anymore.

But the most important change of all is in my self-esteem. For the first time in my life, I can actually say that I like myself and I can accept who I am, with all my faults and my assets.

The Ritalin has changed my life for the better and I will challenge anyone who says that it is not an effective medication for adults to use. I don't want to go back to what my life was like before and I hope that I will be allowed to continue the use of Ritalin for my ADHD.

SONIA D

COMMENT BY DR. WENDER

Sonia D was the first patient I diagnosed as having "minimal brain dysfunction" persisting into adult life. When I first met her and she presented her history, I felt that she was an unhappy woman who had had an exceedingly difficult childhood and had discovered that she felt better when she drank in moderation or took weight pills or stimulant drugs. As we talked about her symptoms and life history, it gradually became clear to me that she was a "minimally brain dysfunctioned" (the old term for ADHD) child grown up. She gave a detailed account of the metamorphoses of her symptoms as she grew older and their response to stimulants, which was atypical—she became calmer, less angry, more trusting. She convinced me that she was what I then thought a real rarity, an "MBD" adult who responded to stimulants as MBD children did. Her history follows. I have now followed her for the past twenty-two years. Her improvement on the overall scale of psychological and occupational functioning was from "moderate to severe impairment" to "slight impairment." Her score on the scale of social adjustment has improved from "moderate-to-severe maladjustment" to "good-to-excellent adjustment."

STATEMENT BY SONIA D

I am a sixty-six-year-old American woman of Russian extraction. I have no physical impairments, and I am reasonably healthy despite being slightly overweight. I have a Ph.D. in Medieval History, I am a member of Phi Beta Kappa, I speak two foreign languages fluently, and have a working knowledge of several others. I am a freelance writer and editor. I have been married for forty years to a medical science professor, and I have had no children.

Because childhood ADHD is so frequently equated with school difficulties, it would seem unlikely that the above-described "achiever" had ever been afflicted with ADHD. I, however, having spent a lifetime in the skin of that individual, have no doubt that I was an ADHD child. Besides the overt "hyperactivity"—including terrible difficulty falling asleep and, once asleep, waking up—I had many of the other signs: impulsiveness, stress intolerance, hot temper, garrulity, bossiness, stubbornness, unpopularity—and I was easily distracted. Moreover, *I am not drastically changed from that child*—except to the extent that I am medicated. Attila the

Hun on tricycle wheels did not undergo a startling trans-
mogrification at the age of thirteen or fourteen. I did not suddenly become a tractable, well-behaved, rational, and controlled adolescent; I merely withdrew. I became a sullen,
fearful, unpopular teenager with periodic episodes of explosive temper. In young adulthood I was unconventional in my
behavior, "pushy" in my dealings with others, and still subject to explosive temper. Since my early forties I have been
medicated with amphetamine, which has given me the control that makes life reasonably peaceful and productive—*but
the child is still there* and, even as a successfully medicated
adult, I have no difficulty identifying with her.

But why, then, did I not fall into the usual life pattern of
one failure after another? I suppose my first advantage was
being bright. Reading—most learning in fact—came easily to
me, and I think I learned how to compensate for my lack of
attention span in one way or another; for instance, somewhere, sometime, early in life, I apparently discovered two
techniques for facilitating any kind of rote learning: (1) I
could concentrate better if my pencil was engaged (taking
notes, scribbling in margins, underlining key words) and (2)
most abstractions could be learned if they could be reduced
to a concrete image (a graph, a chart, an outline, a diagram,
a fanciful cluster of shapes, a technicolor picture on the bland
screen on my brain). Numbers, lists, abstractions, then, never
became *easy*, but at least they became manageable. And, because school was my joy from the first day, I became easily
obsessive about any form of learning.

Another factor could well have been my much maligned
"stubbornness": Each time I was told, "You never finish anything," I responded to the challenge, and the "I'll show you"
attitude kicked in, so that I remember being tenacious about
many tasks that required a good deal of attention span. But
then, I ask, is it truly "attention span" or is it a compulsive,
obsessive desire to compensate for a native distractibility
that wears you out and drives you crazy and makes your day-

to-day existence a painful experience from waking (catastrophe) to sleeping (collapse)? Much of the anguish is trivial, of course: I cannot bear to have someone read over my shoulder or watch me do anything that requires some concentration. I cannot tolerate anyone in the kitchen when I'm preparing a meal. I cannot carry on a conversation or drive if the radio is on. All day long I hear everything and mechanically identify each sound: the mail truck, the cat coming through the swinging pet door, the click in the furnace, the robins in the pyracantha, a sudden shift in the wind. My brain is never on automatic pilot. My husband and I long ago decided that on long trips it made sense for me to do all the driving, since I drove the whole way in any event—whether I was behind the wheel or not. I am incessantly noting and recording facts—important and trifling indiscriminately: the state of the gas gauge, the shaggy brown and white dog on the corner of High Street and the Cornmarket, the position of the town in the relationship to the river, the cop in the white Jaguar squad car in Aberdeen. I'm handy to have around on a second trip to anywhere, because I never forget a place, I know how to get from one side of town to the other, and I'd be a perfect traveling companion if I weren't so habitually uptight, if I didn't gasp *look out!* to the driver, if I didn't bark out orders and directions and become shrill when they weren't carried out to my satisfaction, if I didn't have to stop at the gas station "rest room" so often, if I didn't keep mentioning the funny little rattle in the engine that wasn't there yesterday. . . .

And I cannot bear a wind that lasts longer than three or four hours: It drives me wild and wears me down and sets my teeth on edge and makes me impossible—*more impossible*—to live with. It impinges, intrudes, makes demands on my consciousness, and concentration is then quite out of the question. To put it another way, I feel as if my brain has no filtering system for the massive sensory barrage that relentlessly assails it.

All the other characteristics of ADHD children—impulsiveness, disorderliness, temper, hyperreactivity, unpopularity—I recall well and, in retrospect, I believe they all stem from an overpowering impulse to act. The overriding theme is *urgency*. Everything is urgent. There is no letup. Life is an endless, relentless series of white-knuckle events. All of the miscellaneous dysfunctions (low frustration tolerance, poor planning and judgment, recklessness, disregard for injury, antisocial behavior) are reducible to an urgency that brooks no delay, no postponement, no obstruction to the fulfillment of a necessary goal, which is usually an urge to act. I believe it is a hyperactivation that is not susceptible to reason, to suppression, to socialization, to inhibition—it is a force that is compelling, distressing, and uncontrollable; and it manifests itself in an urgency that cannot be ignored—a kind of "tunnel vision" of life.

Because of a number of chance circumstances, I have had doctors' prescriptions for amphetamine at various times during my life: When I was an undergraduate I consulted the student-health physician for extreme fatigue (we called it my "sleeping sickness" or "hibernation" because it was most prevalent in the fall and winter); she prescribed small doses of amphetamine, which I found fairly miraculous. Parenthetically, all during my undergraduate years I consumed enormous quantities of coffee when I studied. I don't now remember how long I took amphetamine during that period, but I do remember that I was very favorably impressed with the results. When I was in my mid-to-late twenties my husband and I thought we'd like to begin a family; I, however, suffered from endometriosis, a condition that is frequently associated with barrenness. At that time endometriosis was susceptible to a great many tentative—trial and error—courses of treatment, and, having undergone a course of basal-temperature recordings, Cytomel, estrogen, progesterone, myriad combinations thereof, and, as somebody's last resort, D-amphetamine, I was no nearer motherhood than I had ever been—or ever would be. I was, however, about to embark upon a decade of remarkable creativity, productivity, and relative contentment: I explained to my gynecologist that the amphetamine made me feel very good, and he obligingly assured me that there was no harm in my continuing to take the drug. I can no longer remember the trade name of the compound or the dosage, but, as I recall, I had a prescription for 100 tablets, which I had refilled every three months for ten years. I was scrupulous about never exceeding my allotment of drug— perhaps because I sensed that it would be taken away from me if I abused it, perhaps because I never felt a need for more. During that period of purposeful activity, I researched and wrote my first novel, I undertook several major landscaping and decorating projects in the home we had purchased, and I quit smoking—three packages a day. I continued to pursue my intellectual and literary interests, and in 1965 I decided to return to school, this time to earn a degree in History, which I had found to be more broadly appealing than Romance Languages, my undergraduate major. I finished my M.A. in 1968, and in 1970 I successfully passed the qualifying exams for a Ph.D.

In that year the cause of a slow but troublesomely persistent weight gain was traced to moderately severe Gull's disease (underactivity of the thyroid gland). I was—and am still—treated with thyroid hormone, but the amphetamine was judiciously discontinued. It was not a happy decision: While my hypothyroid symptoms—dry skin, edema, hoarse voice, etc.—disappeared, I continued to gain weight, I was depressed, and I was unable to work on my dissertation. After a few months I consulted an internist who specialized in "weight control." He prescribed a reducing diet and issued a prescription for—wonder of wonders—*Didrex*! I eagerly took the drug, followed the diet, lost twenty pounds and was, once again, happy and purposeful. Unfortunately, when I failed to lose more weight, my physician scolded me and withdrew the Didrex, and I ceased to consult him. Again I was depressed, again my weight soared, again I was unable to work on my dissertation. In addition, my alcohol consumption rose sharply and there were severe recurring conflicts with my husband. In January of 1972 I decided to finish my dissertation by June—or die trying. Without telling my metabolics doctor or my husband—who had always objected to my taking Dexedrine—I again appealed to the "weight specialist" I had seen before. Motivated by desperation and reliant on native craftiness, I managed to lose just enough weight to keep the drug coming, and I carefully husbanded whatever excess drug I could squeeze out of my monthly prescription. My credibility with the weight man ran out in May just as I finished the dissertation.

From 1972 (when I received my Ph.D.) until the summer of 1977, I desperately stuffed myself with No-Doz, my weight continued to rise, my inability to make any significant progress on a second novel (begun in 1973) began to be anguishing, my uncontrolled alcohol consumption became debilitating and frankly terrifying, my relationship with my husband deteriorated steadily, I developed a siege mentality, and somewhere within that disordered period I found myself consulting a psychiatrist for depression and frustration at my inability to cope with almost every facet of life—big or small.

Under my psychiatrist's supervision, I began taking Ritalin (later D-amphetamine) in June 1977. In September I finished my novel. (From January 1973 to June 1977, I wrote 250 pages; from June to September 1977, I wrote 400 pages!) I remember feeling that my life had been saved. From that time to this (July 1994) I have taken amphetamine, and if the most reliable proof of the disorder is whether the medication works, then it is clear to me that I do have ADHD because the medication *definitely works*!

The most noticeable effect of both Ritalin and D-amphetamine is a cessation of my normal agitation—physical and mental. The Ritalin has a truly "calming" effect: a serenity that has nothing to do with sedating or euphoria, but seems rather to be a conscious feeling of *control* over irrelevant and intrusive motions and thoughts. Amphetamine, on the other hand, appears to give a purposeful direction, a meaningful channeling to the intensity of one's drive; in other words, it, too, gives *control*, but it appears to be a more dynamic, more decisive control. When I take Ritalin I become aware of the fact that, unmedicated, I habitually clench my teeth and rhythmically move my foot and frequently clutch the arms of my chair; I am aware of these habits by the simple fact of their *absence*. Amphetamine also removes this desultory muscular tension or motion, but it is less noticeable because there may still be activity, but now it has some purpose. In these—admittedly difficult-to-describe—examples I hope to convey the notion that the "good," purposeful activity may be mental as well as physical, because one of the next immediate reactions that I get to either drug is an exquisitely satisfying awareness of the ability to concentrate, to focus, to blot out the massive, indiscriminate sensory input that continuously besieges my brain.

Another striking effect of both drugs is to remove the frightful intensity and urgency of my day-to-day life. This effect is noticeable not only to myself but also to those who know me well and is one of the changes which my husband particularly perceived at an early stage: I become uncharacteristically patient—both with people and things. My "short fuse" is considerably lengthened. I cease to monopolize all conversation. Incidents which once would have driven me to rage and hysteria can now be viewed with a certain objective—*help!*—humor.

In a general way, my interpersonal relationships are also greatly improved. For example, with medication I am free to be warmer, more affectionate; I say *free to be*, because, once my irritability is removed, I no longer have to resent the supposed source of irritation, to wit, whoever is in closest proximity to me. My abandonment of domineeringness is equally dramatic after medication; it is even possible for me to regard my uncharacteristic patience and tolerance with some degree of amazement, for it is still easy for me to imagine vividly how I would normally behave toward the people around me—*outrageously dictatorial and impossibly irascible*. Now, it seems fairly unimportant to insist on my way, on my point of view, on my desires. The life-or-death intensity with which I normally operate is absent, and the potential areas of confrontation appear to be either trivial or childish.

On the negative side, my sleeping problems have not been alleviated: If anything, the sleeping problem is exacerbated by the amphetamine and, as a result, some evenings are most unsatisfactory. If I take my last dose of medication at 3:00 P.M., I may be able to sleep by midnight, but between 8:00 and 12:00 I am sometimes beset by an agitation (rebound hyperexcitability?) that causes me to pace, to become irritable and hostile, to eat compulsively and to consume too much alcohol. Unfortunately, this agitated state is difficult to describe and it is equally difficult to separate out the component parts: How much is ADHD? How much is drug withdrawal? How much is alcohol (which has never had a depressant effect on me until the near "passing out" stage)? During the past twenty-two years I have tried to observe myself and to analyze my actions and responses, and I have come to believe that there is a curious paradox in my behavior: I welcome the control that amphetamine gives me because it permits me to work, because it permits me to maintain decent relationships with others, because it gives me some relief from the terrible intensity of my daily existence; on the other hand, this *controlled* state is not my natural one, for I think that, at heart, I am a kind of incorrigible savage. In other words, my normal ADHD behavior is overlaid by control, but the normal state is, in a strange way, more comfortable, perhaps because it is familiar. In some ways it is a *relief* to return to the state of hyperactivity, irritability, etc. It must be said that I do, after all—even without medication—exert some control over my disorder, however faulty that control may be. Thus, it seems to me that the use of alcohol gives me the license to throw off my inhibitions (my *learned* control) and to revert to my normal (excitable, aggressive) state; that constitutes relief and, of course, enough alcohol permits me to sleep at last. So, then, the end of my day is most always comfortable.

In addition, the positive effects of the drug therapy (concentration, equanimity, domestic tranquility) are so miraculous that it is easy to be stampeded into overoptimism. Alas, there are some negative aspects of your life that do not go away: It's terribly difficult to believe in an "illness" rather than your essential "badness." The tendency to overt self-denigration never really disappears, nor does the guilt: When you are sixty-six your opulently developed sense of guilt is no longer negotiable—especially when you revert to "ADHD behavior." There is a helpless consciousness of transgression *before*, *during* and *after* the event that usually results in a pathetic eagerness to atone, to make amends. When one adds these difficulties to the evening problems, it is obvious that the miracle is not whole. Fractional as it is, however, it is enough to render one—*me*—inalterably grateful. At my age I think I'm dispassionately resigned to living with many of my reactive patterns: guilt, lack of self-esteem, nighttime agitation. These less-than-desirable attributes I can overlook, *if* I can have *control* and *purposeful activity* for the greatest part of my day. A day of serenity and creative accomplishment is a shining reward that makes all "difficulties" pale into insignificance.

GEORGE F

■

COMMENT BY DR. WENDER

George F, forty-nine years old, had been in a Ritalin research study for twelve years. George is adopted, and his family history is unknown. His symptoms at intake were varied and severe. He loved to read but was unable to do much, owing to attention and concentration difficulties. Professionally he had lost numerous jobs because of failure to complete important projects on time, and restlessness and fidgetiness that caused him to (literally) jump around. Extreme disorganization at work and at home were major chronic problems; in fact, he and his wife had separate bedrooms because she can't stand his messiness. His wife described him as chronically irritable, hyperreactive to sounds that don't bother most people, and periodically explosive at home and at work. "The kids never know when or at what he's going to explode."

Emotionally he was mildly depressed, expressed feelings of guilt and inadequacy about letting his family down, but seemed *not to worry* about problems his wife felt he should be worrying about. She was particularly upset about his pattern of making impulsive, inappropriate remarks in social settings that his few close friends put up with and that he didn't understand were inappropriate until much later, if at all.

These severe difficulties continued to plague George even after seven years of psychotherapy. He has been receiving Ritalin, 10 milligrams every three hours four times per day, and after twelve years in our study showed these changes. His overall score on the scale of psychological and occupational functioning improved from "moderate" to "slight impairment," and his score on the scale of social adjustment improved from "moderate to severe maladjustment" to "excellent adjustment."

STATEMENT BY GEORGE F

The controversy surrounding Attention-Deficit Disorder is certainly understandable. Those who haven't experienced it personally or through their children are only aware of the various issues through the simplified media coverage. I know. Even though I have the disorder, it took me a long time to realize that my various struggles could be much more than mere lack of self-discipline. From my understanding of the disorder through the press, I initially felt I didn't suffer from ADHD since I didn't manifest the most obvious symptom: hyperactivity. After all, the other symptoms seem common to everyone to some degree for some of the time. It is hard for most people to comprehend that for a few of us these symptoms are constant and debilitating. It is not a simple disease like the measles or the common cold. We who suffer are so used to the struggle that we are unaware that we are not functioning at a level that others take for granted.

Like most critics, I thought that ADHD was just another fashionable trend in medicine. I felt that taking a magic pill that could change the way your mind works was naive. It was the easy answer for those who were merely avoiding the hard work of learning the skills of concentration, developing good work habits, and simply taking responsibility for one's immaturity. I distrusted drugs in general. Unlike most of my friends in the sixties I didn't take marijuana or LSD. I didn't want to give up what little control I had over my behavior.

For most of my life I held onto the belief that I could change my poor work habits if I could just find the right method of self-discipline. When I began to realize that all the efforts I had made to try to become more efficient, more focused, and more attentive were not working, I reached a level of profound despair. Nothing worked. To make things worse, my wife shared that despair. My marriage and family life were on the verge of failure and I had lost all hope.

Like many adult sufferers of ADHD, it took outside pressure from my spouse to force me to submit to diagnostic tests. Even after I was accepted into the University of Utah's ADHD study group, I had lingering doubts about its worth. I was relieved to have a medical explanation for what I had considered serious personality flaws. However, a lifetime of dashed hopes had left me skeptical of much benefit from a mere pill. I took part in an eight-week study in which I received either Ritalin or a placebo. Neither the doctor nor I knew if I was taking placebos or Ritalin.

The first month was discouraging, since I figured that part of the time I must have been on Ritalin. There was no discernible difference in my behavior that month. I received the second bottle of pills in November 1992. Without much confidence, I took the first pill of this group that evening before I relaxed in my bedroom to read a difficult book that had stymied me for over a month. I didn't feel anything at all from the pill. Somehow I expected a palpable rise in my awareness, a change in my mood, or a bit of a high since Ritalin is, after all, a stimulant. So I forgot about the pill, dismissing it again as worthless. Soon my wife called me to dinner, a little earlier than usual, I thought. I looked at my watch and realized that nearly an hour had passed. As I marked my place in the book I noticed with shock that I had read thirty pages without once losing my train of thought. This may not seem significant to most avid readers but to me it was astonishing. Although I read a great deal, it has always been a struggle for me. Only truly good fiction holds my attention for more than a paragraph. But I had read this particularly turgid nonfiction at a much faster rate than I had ever read any of my favorite books.

I became a believer in the miracle drug Ritalin. Why don't people accept such a possibility when we all know that other drugs are equally amazing? We take aspirin for granted as one of the most effective medicines for pain, but no one has been able to discover how it works. This cheap, simple drug is now being recognized as helpful in controlling heart disease and preventing strokes.

During that next months other subtle changes occurred that were much more apparent to my wife and children. Before I describe the many ways this drug has affected my life, I have to give you an idea what my struggles were like for the previous four decades.

The first clear memory I have of my lack of attention was in fifth grade. I know it was obvious earlier because my mother told me that even my second-grade teacher commented on my "daydreaming." But in fifth grade I remember a specific day when we were reading silently in class about Mexico. As I was reading, I remember feeling anxious that I wouldn't finish the assignment before the class day ended. I kept looking at the clock to see how much time was left and trying to push myself to read faster. I looked at my neighbors' books and noticed they were much farther ahead than I. There was a wonderful photograph of a lush mountainside with a man taking a loaded donkey down a narrow trail. I began to think about being there on that trail, feeling the hot Mexican sun, and hearing the birds in the trees.

Soon I was thinking about the canyon near my home that cuts into the city from the foothills of the Wasatch Mountains. I remembered seeing the Denver-Rio Grande train going past the swimming hole one day of the previous summer. I looked out the window to see if the weather was good enough to go down there that day right after school. My teacher noticed me gazing out the window and asked me if I had finished already. She became angry when I said no and took me out into the hall. She gave me a stern lecture about my lack of "stick-to-itiveness" and embarrassed me deeply. I remember vowing to never let that happen ever again. But, despite all my efforts, it occurred over and over again, even through college. Every time I caught my mind wandering from the text, I would try to force myself to focus. It never worked. In minutes my mind would be on another track. It was apparent that the harder I tried, the more anxious I became, which inevitably caused me to think about not getting finished and imagining the consequences instead of focusing. It never occurred to me that there was anything I could do besides vowing to learn how to change my bad habits. But none of the study techniques I tried seemed to help. I generally approached my work in a state of panic, spending late hours trying to catch up, and developing a chronic case of diarrhea.

All through school I never finished a single textbook. I specifically recall being desperate about chemistry. Despite my intense determination to do well, I was only able to read two of the seventeen chapters assigned for that year. I still managed to get a C in the class. In most of my classes, I survived purely by my wits. Fortunately, my memory for facts has been phenomenal and compensated for my inability to focus on my reading. Taking notes was a disaster since it got in the way of my listening. Since I got good grades, my parents never worried about my work and never pushed me to do better. They were just happy that I wasn't a poor student like my three brothers. They didn't suspect that I was having difficulties.

They didn't have to push me because I already did so myself, mercilessly. I would consistently stay up to one or two in the morning to work on assignments which should have taken half the time. I would come to school exhausted, often with my work unfinished. Teachers regularly gave me good grades on my incomplete papers because it was obvious that I understood the assignments. Report cards would usually comment on my incompletes, that I was capable of doing much better.

Because I loved literature, my favorite class was English. I eventually majored in English in college. I often came early to my favorite high school English teacher's class to talk about what we were reading in class and about other fiction as well. Despite my constant lack of full preparation I would still find time to read other things. She told me near the end of the year that I had a wonderful mind for literature but it was too bad that I didn't work hard enough. I remember thinking that I couldn't possibly work any harder.

One symptom I never had to any great degree was hyperactivity. Perhaps if I had, my ADHD would have been recognized earlier in life. Of course, in the 1950s and early 1960s hyperactivity was not yet considered anything more than poor behavior. The most I would do was bounce my leg rapidly in my chair or tap my pencil. This would irritate my parents, and later my wife, but I was only admonished to quit doing it. I could sit at my desk without jumping up and running around like other ADHD kids.

However, I was very impulsive. When my mind wandered away from the immediate tasks at hand I would think of other things I needed to do and drop what I was doing and pursue the distracting interest. Too many things had the capability to distract me from the more crucial tasks. In a perverse way this was often beneficial to my education. For instance, whenever I read an unfamiliar word, I would immediately look it up in the dictionary. Words have always fascinated me. However, once in the dictionary, I would look up synonyms, antonyms, and the etymologies of the word I was researching. Often the simple goal of looking up a single word would take half an hour or more. Although my vocabulary and spelling skills grew to be impressive, I wouldn't be able to finish reading anything within a reasonable time. Distractions would also benefit my later interest in architecture. The tendency to go off on a different angle would aid my designs because my divergent thinking often led to unique ideas and other possibilities that could not be predicted in a strictly linear approach. Unfortunately, precious time would be lost and I would have to work long hours to synthesize these ideas into a coherent whole. Usually this would leave me exhausted and many of the details needed to complete the design would be poorly thought out.

Usually the content of my reading would stimulate related but diverging thoughts. This helped me to gain better insights about literature through analogy. Mention of an unfamiliar event, topic, or person would drive me to my encyclopedia in another time-consuming digression.

This was also particularly noticeable in my speech. If I were talking with someone about some idea I would often veer off the track in mid-sentence with a related point. This would generally lead to yet another diverging explanation until I would lose all sense of my original direction. While listening to others, I would be thinking of my next thought, which I feared would vanish before I had time to respond. I would blurt it out before the speaker had a chance to finish his point.

Since my mother also had this annoying tendency, our conversations were particularly chaotic. She would complain that I didn't have a clutch on my tongue, that my speech would jerk into motion before I engaged my mind. Of course, her habit of finishing my sentences for me while I was searching for the right words drove me crazy.

Needless to say, my social skills did not develop in a normal manner. Many people would gradually drift away from me while I tried to talk to them. I tended to keep quiet whenever I met new people. Parties were never much fun. I was particularly uncomfortable when I met anyone who spoke with grace and ease. By the time I graduated from high school I was so resentful of the popular students that I was becoming bitter, sarcastic, and deeply depressed. I not only had not gained any confidence in myself but I began to lose hope that I would ever be able to perform the tasks necessary for success in any field that I wanted to pursue. When teachers or employers would give me instructions, my mind would often be racing along unproductive directions. I would try to take extensive notes during and after instructions but they were inevitably chaotic and difficult to read.

My attempts to organize my work led me to try many different techniques that would have been effective for the average person. But they rarely worked for me. I would be thinking of too many things at the same time and be frustrated about learning how to make priorities. Despite the many files I organized, I would usually lose some crucial bit of information and waste my energy trying to recover it. I became fanatical about having all the information I needed to finish a project. If I didn't know an answer to some matter, its importance would grow into an obsession. I grew more and more unable to make simple decisions.

Despite all my problems I managed to receive a degree in English Literature and later a Masters in Architecture. After I got my professional license, I began to believe that maybe I had grown out of my bad habits. However, they continued to persist and even got worse.

Becoming an adult did not end my ADHD. Of course, I didn't realize that my problem had a neurological basis. I continued to feel depressed about the pervasive nature of my problems. Nothing seemed to work for me. In twenty years of professional practice, I did not advance to the level of income, performance, and ability that I knew I was capable of achieving if I could only work productively. I resented my colleagues who did much better than I, those whose design abilities were less than mine. Of course, I rationalized; they knew how to use the system better than I. I became very adept at finding excuses for losing jobs, blaming others for my failures.

I turned this onto my wife as well. My negativity almost destroyed my marriage. I blamed her for being too difficult, too demanding. I realize now how badly I abused her trust and love. Even though I knew she had the right to expect me to be home when I said I would be, my inability to predict how long a project would take drove her to despair. It was so hard to keep my work timely and give her and our children the attention they deserved. My frustration with work left me irritable with my family. Often, I would explode in unpredictable anger. Thankfully, they kept their faith in me long enough for me to discover the possibility that I had ADHD.

It would be an exaggeration to claim that my life has changed overnight into a wonderful dream since I have been on Ritalin, but the long nightmare is at last over. Although I still have a lot to relearn about organization, time management, social skills, and obsession with detail, I no longer feel despair or anxiety. I can now make reasonable estimates about the time necessary to complete projects and finish them without resorting to long anxiety-ridden nights. My relationships with my employers and fellow workers have improved significantly. I'm more cooperative and attentive to their needs. Architecture has now become the delightful profession I had long ago wished it would be. I no longer drag myself to work late and exhausted because I stayed up late trying to catch up.

Ritalin literally saved my marriage and my relationships with my children and close friends. I pay attention to them without getting defensive, critical, or insensitive. The last twelve years with my wife have been a marvelous restoration of our initial love for each other. We share much more time with each other and her trust in me continues to grow. I no longer keep her waiting up for me past the time I have told her I would be home. I don't make us late for movies or parties because I always know where I leave my keys now. She tells me her feelings now without fear that I will criticize them as irrational, which they never were.

Distractions still occur, of course, but I do not impulsively respond to them. I have limited my nonarchitectural interests to those that are important to me. I have enjoyed researching a particular social problem (not ADHD) that I have deeply cared about for twenty years. My writing about it has received recognition from the international press and a growing audience of those intimately involved in it. One of the rewards of this effort has been several opportunities to travel and speak to the public. Last year I went all the way to Melbourne, Australia, to speak to the Victorian Parliament, several other groups, and to the press.

This is amazing to me since I had never been comfortable speaking about ideas for fear that I would make a complete fool of myself. I can confidently speak to many people at once and maintain a coherent direction without confusing them with digressions. This is immensely satisfying after a lifetime of being unable to express myself.

As I said at the start, I can understand the lack of acceptance of ADHD as a neurological disorder and the effectiveness of its treatment through a mere drug. Unless someone has gone through the agony of my experiences, it is difficult to accept. I can only hope that critics can suspend judgment about this until more evidence is gathered. I am confident that it will be appreciated in the near future and that the medical profession will finally recognize the validity of the diagnosis and its treatment. Scientific revolutions have often been dismissed as false, even blasphemous. Galileo, Darwin, Pasteur, and many others had suffered the outrageous criticism that ADHD researchers are now receiving from reactionary groups like the Church of Scientology. For the sake of the thousands of sufferers of Attention-Deficit Hyperactivity Disorder, both children and adults, I hope that sympathy and understanding will soon prevail over the hysterical forces of ignorance. They deserve the right to experience a life relatively free from confusion and despair.

COMMENT BY SPOUSE OF GEORGE F

It's always been hard to put my finger on exactly what was so difficult about living with George. By all standards, he was the ideal mate: he worked hard, was faithful, wasn't abusive, was highly intelligent, and extremely good-looking.

My complaints were those of every married woman: he was uncommunicative; he kept me waiting for hours; he didn't care about my feelings; our ways of managing money and disciplining children were diametrically opposed; etc.

The problems were run-of-the-mill but abnormal in the sense that they were extreme and unrelenting: for example, he would estimate that he had three or four hours of work before coming home but it turned out to be *eighteen* hours, an "all-nighter."

My emotional history made me very vulnerable to someone not showing up. I would be in a state of panic for hours. Even though I told George how much I suffered when he kept me waiting, he never changed his behavior. I could never count on him to be on time, to help me with decisions or with the children. He just could not attend to his inner world and to the rest of the problems of living.

One night we came home at midnight and our thirteen-year-old son was playing catch at the corner. I yelled at him to come home. He didn't. I asked George to deal with the problem and he got furious with me for yelling, thereby disturbing the neighbors.

An angry tone of voice always irritated him. Once he got mad because the sound of my daughter chewing croutons irritated him. It took hours of discussion for me to convince him to be reasonable. I thought that I was the one who was lacking in relating and communicating skills. This eroded my self-esteem.

His behavior was unpredictable, impulsive and almost completely unresponsive to outside influence. Raising my voice, confrontation, asserting my needs, explaining, getting angry, moving out twice, not only failed to get my needs met but resulted in his asserting that I was the "bad guy."

A typical scenario occurred the summer our twelve-year-old daughter was in a recital at a music camp in St. George [Utah]. After the five-hour drive George arrived rather di-

sheveled and his appearance caused our daughter some embarrassment. The next day we were attending the recital and
after examining the program, George assumed that he would
have time to go get a haircut before Jennifer's turn. After
twenty-five years of marriage I knew that it was useless to
advise him not to do this. So he went and of course missed
her performance. After everything was over, he insisted that
she go to the piano and play the piece for him so that he
could get a picture. She was upset and uncooperative and
George was irritated.

As my psychiatrist put it, being around George was like
"having to walk on eggshells."

The stresses of any change in his routine (like a vacation)
exacerbated his condition: Once he lost a contact lens while
taking it out at dusk at a windswept roadside stop; another
time, he left his wallet on top of the car and lost it, thus
ruining our skiing holiday. In France, he got so angry when
a driver tailgated and passed us that he had to follow the
driver and do the same thing.

He was not a mean person, and as long as I left him alone
and didn't need anything from him, he was fine and quite
mellow. He couldn't tolerate the mildest stresses of family
life. The unremitting nature of his impulsive and irrational
behavior and the inability to grow and develop into a fully
sharing partner are the factors that made our problems different from the usual marital difficulties.

After twenty-five years of marriage plus three years of
courtship, and after George had been in psychoanalysis for
seven years, I was ready to die: I had gotten nowhere in my
various careers and I couldn't love the man to whom I had
committed so much of my life.

And then one final crisis and the miracle of the ADHD
diagnosis and the Ritalin cure occurred.

I had left my job when George had managed to hang on to
a job for two years. Our daughter had been accepted at Yale
and then, once again, he was laid off (the seventeenth time
in eighteen years).

This time, finally, I came to the certain conclusion that my husband suffered from a neurological problem. It had become imperative that he be correctly diagnosed and somehow taught to adapt to his handicap.

My conversations with George, like everyone else's, were difficult to impossible. Either he said nothing but yes or no to questions that would normally require elaboration, or he would go on and on and on about whatever topic had grabbed his interest at the moment, with no desire for input from the person who was listening to him. If I expressed disinterest even with just a look, he would become defensive.

I concluded that his disorder was very much analogous to being deaf as he seemed to not perceive other human beings' nonverbal language and expectations.

The changes in George's behavior in the twelve years he's been on Ritalin are as hard to describe as it is to describe the disorder. They are very subtle but the children and I can tell as soon as he opens his mouth whether or not he's taken the medication. Mainly, he isn't so defensive; he doesn't get his dander up at every little thing that doesn't go his way. He listens, and he shuts up when he perceives that no one wants to listen to him. He is more spontaneous and invites me to share in some of his activities. He is accepting when I decline.

He has always worked very hard and was phenomenally energetic. He never seemed to tire. Whereas before he dissipated his energy going from one project to another, focusing on his interests rather than on results, now he completes project after project: gardening, remodeling the house, writing, and of course his professional duties.

In summary, I really can't find the words to express what a difference George's treatment with Ritalin has made in my life. The very first pill was more effective than twenty-eight years of love and patience and understanding and seven years of psychotherapy.

I have a Master's degree in neurophysiology and have worked for nearly thirty years in neuroscience and as a teacher of disturbed adolescents. I am an expert on Freud. I would never have believed that a drug could have such a profound effect on someone's behavior.

First of all, I thought that a drug's action would be too global to be effective. Secondly, I thought George's problems stemmed from having been brought up in a dysfunctional family and that he needed to learn new behaviors. Now I am convinced that Ritalin affects the firing of neurons such that perception of the outside world is different than it is without the medication.

BRUCE C

■

COMMENT BY DR. WENDER

Bruce C was a fifty-four-year-old teacher and sports coach who left his job after more than a dozen years at the same school because of an accumulation of complaints both at school and in the community. He described himself as having been very restless and inattentive during elementary school, where he had a difficult time learning and was a "troublemaker." When he was four years old he told his parents that his brother had drowned, "just to get a rise out of them." As a six or seven year old he got annoyed and broke all the windows in his father's car. He had very low feelings of self-esteem. Not only was he a recognized problem in the school but his father was the town drunk. His Parents' Rating Scale score was 22 (over the 99th percentile—see Appendix). There was a family history of alcoholism. Both his parents, his brother, and one sister were alcoholics, and the patient said he would have become one too had he not vowed (successfully) not to drink much. At the time of his entrance into the research study, he had just left his teaching job and was in the process of looking unsuccessfully for another job. Under this pressure his ADHD symptoms had become more severe. He was having chronic difficulty with his wife and was estranged from his two older children. During the placebo and drug trials he showed no response to placebo and yet had a marked beneficial effect from Ritalin. The dose was eventually standardized at 90 milligrams a day (15 milligrams every two and half hours, six times per day). He has been continued on the drug for ten years without any signs at all of the development of tolerance. His overall score on the scale of psychological and occupational functioning improved from "moderate-to-severe maladjustment" to "slight maladjustment." His score on the scale of social adjustment improved from "moderate-to-severe maladjustment" to "excellent adjustment."

COMMENT BY SPOUSE OF BRUCE C

When I met and started dating Bruce in the 1960s, he was in the U.S. Army. I dated him and got to know him pretty well over the next year. I also knew his parents, and his four brothers and sisters. As I got to know his family better I noticed that most of his family members were very "quick tempered," and seemed to act quite impulsively. While dating Bruce, I lived with his sister, while we were both in the process of getting a divorce. One of the most common examples of his sister's behavior is that she never allowed enough time to get ready for work and almost always ended up throwing either the iron or her clothes across the room and bursting into tears and usually blaming whatever, or whomever, she could. The family thought of themselves as "outspoken." I thought they acted without much thought or common sense. In most circumstances Bruce and I got along quite well. We were not in very many stressful situations, even though I did observe that Bruce had a "quick temper," usually directed at the "idiots" on the road that didn't know how to drive. He was also very sensitive and thought people were talking about him, but often they would be, to comment on his "quick tempered" behavior.

All of the C family liked to consume alcohol, and this habit seemed to enhance all of these negative behaviors. Both of his parents drank regularly, his father daily, his mother usually all weekend. All of his family drank more than occasionally, and Bruce's only brother and one sister have been in several programs for alcoholics. Bruce quit shortly after our marriage, or I'm positive we never would have made a life together. Whenever under the influence it was common to have verbal and physical confrontations dancing at a local club. Bruce felt like the bartender was not putting the amount of alcohol he should have been putting, so he took a drink of it and threw it across the room into the jukebox. When the waitress came over, he told her he wanted a drink with some alcohol now.

The thing the C's were most successful at was excusing each other's and their own behavior, always claiming that if "they hadn't screwed up" or if "he would have shut up" or if "she would have just did what she should have," then they wouldn't have become angry or lost control. This behavior bothered me a lot. However, Bruce and I decided not to consume much alcohol, which helped greatly, and until after we married in 1967, I didn't observe this behavior very often. Since Bruce was and is a very intelligent and caring person, it seemed I could overlook the other behavior, and like every woman in the world, I thought he would improve with time—Bruce didn't. I observed very belligerent, impulsive behavior whenever a near-crisis situation would come up—for example, arriving in a large West Coast city and having Bruce behind the wheel and trying to survive his outrageous out-of-control behavior when he couldn't find the address, which was always. He would, as I called it, pull his big "R&R" (ranting and raving) until I could visualize somehow getting him out of the car and then either running over him or driving off and leaving him and never seeing him again.

There are literally hundreds of similar examples over the years. Instead of carrying out either of the examples I just used, I chose to distance myself from Bruce. By the early 1970s we had four small children. I spent a lot of my next years keeping every stressful situation from Bruce that I could, covering for the kids so they didn't make Daddy angry, and even though Bruce was quite successful at blaming me for his behaviors, I tried never to let him do it to the kids and handled everything that I could alone. I learned to resent and feel unhappy and lonely most of the time. I tried to invite family or friends to our home when Bruce had to work, because when people were visiting were the times he would always manage to have a reason to be out of control and usually yell at me and usually throw something or just be generally rude. Every time we had events we had to go to I would try just to leave Bruce home. My salvation, so to speak, was that along with his working full-time and part-time, when he was home he wanted to be left alone and spent all of his time at home watching TV.

Bruce spent over a dozen years teaching. At this job and his part-time job, even though he was always very qualified, he continued over the years to have personality conflicts with unruly kids and their parents, and though very educated and knowing what he wanted to communicate to people, it never worked out. Bruce was the "most unlucky," "misunderstood" person in the world, and he always ended up losing his temper and letting the other person know the problem belonged to them, and that they were idiots. Bruce went through hell, because of these problems, and finally over the years Bruce even started realizing as I did that these were "his problems." Finally in the late 1980s, he was given the choice to resign or be fired from teaching, and he resigned. He felt very "picked on" and had a very hard year out of work and found it impossible to get another job that was very impressive, or paid very much. We were barely staying married and were both very unhappy, but with eight children we didn't have too many choices. I am positive if Bruce hadn't gotten into the ADHD study, I would have divorced him.

About his situation in life. One day while he was listening to the radio he heard someone talking about a federal study in ADHD. They talked about the symptoms and effects this could have on someone's life—Bruce quickly called me to listen and asked me who this might sound like. It described Bruce *exactly*. We got on the phone and made an appointment and went in.

The first two weeks Bruce was on Ritalin I could tell a great change in him. Instead of him barely being able to concentrate on one conversation or one telephone call, he could watch TV and listen in on my phone conversation, which I never had to worry about all of the years I knew him. I found him being able to communicate with the kids and follow through with reasonable discipline. One son commented that he liked Dad better before he "knew what was going on" because now he would follow through when he grounded them or whatever he was doing with them. Soon he could even talk to our oldest son with no tempers flaring, and being aware of how he would have reacted earlier in life. For the first time I dared to count on Bruce to help me with our now large family. I slowly started to confide in him about a few things, and found I could even vent a little anger about my life.

There is *no*, none, no way that ours would still be an existing family if it weren't for this medication and the counseling therapy that has gone along with it. I feel that Bruce's improvement is both medication and behavior modification. However, if a crisis of any dimension comes up when he hasn't had his meds, we have a very painful recall of past times. Bruce is different in almost every way. He has always wanted to be someone we could count on and talk to and have those he cares about and works with value and respect his opinions. This happens often now.

Bruce works for the government doing a job that is very detailed and takes more concentration than he ever could have had anytime prior to this study. He stayed totally away from computers, because they drove him crazy. Now at his job Bruce helped change his department over to computers, and is a very well-respected, valued employee. He contributes ideas and several of his ideas have been incorporated as policy. His communication skills have improved drastically at home and at work. Several years ago Bruce went back to a state university and received an advanced degree and updated his teaching certificate, and while working full-time and going to school full-time graduated with a 4.0 in his major and a 3.7 overall. Bruce seems to have gained a lot of confidence and isn't afraid people won't respect or listen to him. His life has improved in every way possible.

7

Finding Help

■

FINDING HELP FOR THE CHILD
WITH ADHD

■

As I have discussed, frequently problems that may be related to Attention-Deficit Hyperactivity Disorder are often first recognized in the school by teachers, guidance counselors, or psychologists who call the parents' attention to these problems. In some instances—particularly in these days when knowledge of ADHD has spread widely—parents themselves begin to suspect their child has behavioral problems beyond the normal range. I wish to emphasize again that, in either case, in order to determine the probable cause of the child's difficulties, parents must consult a physician who is knowledgeable about the entire range of children's physical and emotional problems, including ADHD. A thorough diagnostic evaluation is essential before beginning any treatment plan.

The following kinds of physicians are most likely to be acquainted with the problems of ADHD: child psychiatrists, pediatricians, and pediatric neurologists. What are their backgrounds? All physicians attend four years of medical school, have one year of postgraduate general medical training (internship), and then receive additional training in their specialty. Child psychiatrists receive two years training in adult psychiatry and two in child psychiatry; they are then eligible to take specialized "board" examinations.

All psychiatrists, like all other physicians, must continue to attend courses and engage in other academic activities to maintain their medical licenses, and must be recertified by the specialized board periodically.

Child psychiatrists are best qualified to evaluate and treat ADHD in children because their training is broad and encompasses the diagnosis and treatment not only of ADHD, but of all psychiatric disorders of childhood, including those that may occur together with ADHD and those that may be mistaken for it. Most child psychiatrists now recognize that many of the disorders they see are the result of genetic and biological causes and are best treated with medication. However, child psychiatrists are also experienced in evaluation and treatment of psychological problems that accompany or result from childhood ADHD and are trained in the psychological treatment of these disorders.

Pediatricians and pediatric neurologists also treat ADHD and other childhood problems. Pediatricians have two years of post-internship training in the medical disorders of children and adolescents that includes some, usually brief, training in child psychiatry. Pediatric neurologists are pediatricians who have subspecialized in children's diseases of the nervous system. Many years ago ADHD was thought to be due to brain damage or neurological malfunction, and ADHD children where often seen by pediatric neurologists. They too have had relatively brief training in child psychiatry.

Many pediatricians and family practitioners treat a large number of ADHD patients. There are several reasons for this. Often parents with an ADHD child who have been referred to a psychiatrist will not go, believing that psychiatrists treat only very seriously disturbed children. They fear that accepting such a referral would mean that their child is much sicker than they had realized. Sometimes pediatricians or general physicians will treat ADHD patients because they feel they can handle it themselves or because they feel there are no competent child psychiatrists in the community. Finally, there are simply too few child psychiatrists to treat the number of children in the community who require help.

Pediatricians and family physicians vary tremendously in their skill and handling of diagnosis, drug management, and psychological assistance of children with ADHD. Some have little training in treating behavior problems while others can treat most routine cases and are quick to refer more complicated problems to child psychiatrists. Yet others who do not recognize the possible complexity of ADHD approach all kinds of ADHD children in the same way, and thus risk providing inadequate treatment.

Mental health workers such as psychologists, nurse practitioners, social workers, and counselors are frequently the first professionals contacted after a referral for evaluation. Although many are experienced at recognizing ADHD and skilled in the treatment of some of the associated symptoms and behavioral problems, they cannot perform the complex medical evaluation necessary nor can they prescribe medication. Child and adolescent psychiatrists often work with such professionals in the management of the child with ADHD. If available, such a collaborative approach can often be very useful.

FINDING HELP FOR THE ADULT WITH ADHD

■

The physicians best qualified to treat ADHD in adults are psychiatrists. They are trained in the biological and psychological causes of psychiatric disorders and the biological and psychological treatment of them. Other physicians who sometimes treat adult ADHD are pediatricians (who occasionally follow their patients into adolescence and early adulthood), family practitioners, and internists. Their background in psychiatry has generally been minimal. The psychiatrist, particularly one who has focused on biological psychiatry and the treatment of psychiatric disorders with medication, is therefore the physician best suited for the job. Not only has he or she been trained to manage ADHD, but is able to diagnose and treat other conditions that may accompany or mimic it. Additionally, the psychiatrist can recognize the remaining ADHD symptoms that did not respond to medical treatment, the maladjustments that ADHD patients suffer because of their disorder—difficulties with their partner or their job—and which are due to other psychiatric problems. The psychiatrist is in the best position to refer the adult ADHD patient for further treatment as needed: couple therapy, family therapy, or vocational training. Should both a parent and a child need psychiatric treatment, whether for ADHD or another disorder, if at all possible separate psychiatrists should be consulted.

FINDING A PSYCHIATRIST

Having determined that the best specialist to treat either childhood or adult ADHD is a psychiatrist, what is the next step? The best place to start is to request a referral from one's family physician or pediatrician. One can also inquire of the state or district branch of the American Psychiatric Association (APA). These days one will also have to inquire of one's insurance company for a list of psychiatrists on their panel. These inquiries will yield the names of several psychiatrists practicing in the community. The caller can ask whether the psychiatrist is board certified or not. However, none of these sources provide an evaluation of the psychiatrist's skill or areas of specialization. Another way to locate specialists in the treatment of ADHD is to contact the department of psychiatry in nearby university medical schools. In particular, ask the child and adolescent psychiatry department if they have specialized treatment for ADHD or behavior disorders, and the adult department if they have a research or treatment clinic for mood disorders (which include depression, manic-depression, and, usually, ADHD). Such clinics not only conduct research but also evaluate new drugs and train young psychiatrists in the diagnosis and treatment of these disorders. The level of expertise in these clinics is usually high, and they are often able to recommend not only their own staff but also psychiatrists practicing in the community.

If the university medical school does not have such a clinic, it is sometimes helpful to ask whether any of the senior staff or members of the department of psychiatry see private patients. However, physicians associated with medical schools are not necessarily better trained than physicians in the community. The odds are greater that a physician chosen at random is well trained if associated with a medical school, but it is important to emphasize strongly that there are many excellent psychiatrists who are not. I refer patients to such psychiatrists all the time; some of them are in private practice and some are in private clinics that specialize in the drug treatment of psychiatric disorders.

Many communities have community mental health clinics that are supported by federal and state funding and offer psychiatric services on a sliding-fee scale. Philosophies of the clinic and the expertise of their psychiatric staff vary considerably. In some, evaluation is done by nonpsychiatrists. In others, all evaluations are conducted or reviewed by psychiatrists. Community health clinics have the advantage of lower fees, but the prospective patient must still ask the questions about their training that we have mentioned in discussing other physicians who treat ADHD.

After selecting a physician, and after the initial consultation, it is also appropriate to ask how frequent the visits will be and how much they will cost. Should any doubts trouble the parent or adult patient, it is always proper to request another consultation or evaluation. Once treatment has begun, if the treatment prescribed is not working after a reasonable period of time, say six months, another consultation should be requested. Finally, it must be remembered that all problems are not solvable in all people, adults or children.

I should warn both parents who suspect their children of having ADHD as well as prospective patients seeking help for what they think is ADHD that they must anticipate some close questioning by the physician. Some physicians will be cautious of parental or self-diagnosis of ADHD, since ADHD is being diagnosed on a larger and larger scale and many patients are mistakenly seeking help for a variety of other psychiatric difficulties that they have attributed to ADHD. Be prepared for, and willing to accept, reasonable questions from the evaluating mental health worker.

THE EVALUATION PROCEDURE AND TREATMENT FOR THE CHILD WITH ADHD

In order to give parents some idea of what a good evaluation for ADHD involves, I have listed below the diagnostic techniques usually employed. This summary is not meant to serve as a checklist, but to convey to the parent some awareness of what adequate evaluation includes. I will also mention procedures that might be unnecessary or overly expensive in terms of the information they are likely to yield. From a competent evaluation and treatment plan, the parent can expect the following.

1. A detailed psychological history of the child will be requested, preferably from both parents. The purpose of the history is to determine the child's strengths and weaknesses, his

assets and deficiencies, by finding out how he has gotten along with his parents, his siblings, his peers, and his teachers. The history will not be limited simply to establishing the presence or absence of the symptoms listed in the DSM-IV criteria for ADHD (reprinted in the Appendix), but will include those discussed in this book. The physician will want to know about all behavioral symptoms that might indicate other psychiatric disorders that resemble ADHD or that might occur together with ADHD and require special treatment. Such symptoms may be those of anxiety, depression, alcohol and substance abuse, and others; they are described more fully in the Appendix.

2. A review of biological factors that may be related to ADHD and a medical history will be undertaken. Such questions as the following will be asked: Is there a history of psychiatric disorders among the child's relatives? Did the mother drink, smoke, or use drugs during pregnancy? Were there any problems with delivery? Has the child had any experiences that may have affected the brain, including infection or head injury?

3. Reports from the school will be requested to determine the child's performance, both academically and socially. These may be given over the telephone, by written report, or with standardized questionnaires filled out by the child's teacher. Questionnaires are not only useful in diagnosis, but also, when the child is being treated, can serve as an excellent method of determining the amount of improvement in academic achievement and social behavior that are produced by treatment.

4. Parents will be asked to fill out questionnaires. These may be broad in scope to evaluate general psychological problems of childhood or specialized to measure only ADHD symptoms. Like the teacher questionnaires, the parent questionnaires can be used to evaluate the progress produced by treatment.

5. Psychological tests may be required. If the child has

learning problems, educational tests are usually obtained to measure both intelligence and level of academic achievement. The goal is to determine if the child's difficulty is due to some degree of intellectual slowness or whether, despite the presence of normal or above-average intelligence, there are difficulties in reading, spelling, or math—that is, signs of Learning Disorders. Neurological tests are not generally needed unless there is a suspicion of epilepsy or other neurological disease. In other words, it is highly unlikely that specialized X rays or electroencephalograms will be required.

6. Laboratory tests of attention may be obtained. Two relatively new tests are being used to measure the degree of inattention, distractibility, and impulsivity. The first is the Continuous Performance Test, in which the subject responds to patterns of flashing light. Depending on which letters are presented on a video monitor, the subject does or does not push a button. The second is the Test of Variable Attention, in which the subject responds to different shapes on the video monitor under conditions similar to the Continuous Performance Test. ADHD children show impairment of performance as compared to normal children, with their performance often improving after medication is administered. However, neither test can prove or disprove a diagnosis of ADHD; their usefulness in the treatment of patients remains to be shown.

7. An interview with the child will be conducted. Sometimes symptoms of other psychiatric disorders are present and may not become evident until the physician talks with the child. Not all problems with attention and behavior are the result of ADHD; other problems may look like ADHD or occur together with ADHD, and the child may be misdiagnosed and receive partial or incorrect treatment. The parents may be unaware of anxiety, depression, and many other conditions affecting the child because the child is not forthcoming and does not report these problems spontaneously. Often, the physician may, with tact and time, uncover these

masked problems and thus be able to provide specific treatments.

8. Time will be spent with the child and with the parents explaining the child's specific problems in ways that both can understand. Time will also be spent with the parents discussing management techniques useful with an ADHD child; management strategies are discussed in this book.

In follow-up visits the parent can expect the following procedures:

1. To determine the effects of medication on behavior, the physician will request feedback from the parents and usually from the school as well. School reports are particularly important because the teacher is observing the child in the areas in which the child has the most difficulty: performing schoolwork, staying on tasks and finishing them, and getting along with other children.

2. To determine the amount of medication, the physician will probably vary the dosage to see the extent to which symptoms can be controlled. The general principle is to increase the dose until either the symptoms are controlled or the side effects become unpleasant.

3. To determine the frequency of dosage, the physician will ask the parent to observe the child (best on weekends) to determine how long each dose of medication lasts and therefore how frequently the dose must be given.

THE EVALUATION PROCEDURE
AND TREATMENT FOR
THE ADULT WITH ADHD

■

From a competent evaluation and treatment plan, an adult patient can expect the following:

1. The presence of a partner, parent, or friend will be re-

quested. This other person should be one who can help in the discussion of the patient's past and current problems. As I have mentioned repeatedly, the adult with ADHD who is entering evaluation and treatment does not fully recognize the extent of his signs and symptoms. When giving a history, the patient will be asked to cite as many concrete instances as he can of his difficulties in functioning in each of the seven areas of the Utah Diagnostic Criteria (listed in the Appendix). The presence of a person who knows the patient well may give a much richer, more detailed and accurate picture of the patient's past and current functioning.

2. The patient's development in childhood and adolescence will be reviewed. How did he get along with siblings, schoolmates, parents, and parenting figures? What was his academic performance like in elementary school, high school, and higher education?

3. If Learning Disorders are present, the physician will want to obtain the same psychoeducational tests that are used in evaluating children.

4. A history will be requested concerning adult interpersonal relationships with friends, spouse, partners, and colleges.

5. A history will be requested of drug or alcohol use.

6. Questions will be asked about symptoms of other psychiatric disorders that resemble ADHD or that may occur together with ADHD and require special treatment. As in the case with children, these symptoms may relate to anxiety, depression, or other disorders as listed in Chapter 6 and the Appendix.

7. A private conversation between the physician and the patient will be held because there are many issues that the patient may be reluctant to discuss in front of his partner, including other symptoms, feelings he cannot mention, and some life experiences, such as outside relationships. For similar reasons, the physician will probably want to talk to the

partner individually to question him or her about matters each might feel uncomfortable discussing in the presence of the patient.

8. If ADHD is diagnosed, a treatment program will be proposed that will consist of what the physician will provide medically and the steps he or she believes the patient should take psychologically. The latter will partially be determined by the extent of the patient's response to medical treatment.

On follow-up, the patient can expect the following:

1. The physician will want to know both from the patient and the partner how effective specific doses of the medication are in reducing or controlling the symptoms and how long they last. This is essential in determining the best dose and the best frequency of its administration. Often the treating physician will use a checklist or behavior rating scale to measure the patient's symptoms on a week-to-week basis.

2. As with children, if psychological problems remain after medical treatment, the physician may either decide to provide psychotherapy and training himself or may recommend referral elsewhere for such training or for couple or marital therapy.

OTHER SOURCES OF HELP

■

C.H.A.D.D. (Children and Adults with Attention-Deficit Disorders) is the national and international nonprofit parents' support organization for children and adults with ADHD and can inform you of organizations and C.H.A.D.D. groups in your locality. Their address is 499 NW 70th Ave., Suite 308, Plantation, FL 33317; telephone (305) 587-3700; fax (305) 587-4599. Learning Disabilities Association of America, 4156 Library Road, Pittsburgh, PA 15234; telephone (412) 341–1515 is another resource. The American Academy of Child and Adolescent Psychiatry publishes a series of leaflets, called

Facts for Families, that covers a wide range of childhood problems. They will also direct you to your local branch for referral: 3615 Wisconsin Ave, NW, Washington DC 20016; telephone (800) 333-7636. A book that may be of help to the professional is Paul H. Wender, M.D., *Attention-Deficit Hyperactivity in Adults* (Oxford University Press, New York, 1995). It is a book written primarily for the professional, but the lay reader may find the descriptions of symptoms, the rating scales (for determining the presence of ADHD in childhood), and the detailed discussion of medication particularly useful.

APPENDIX

Diagnostic Criteria: Diagnosis of ADHD and Related Disorders in Childhood and Adulthood

■

DIAGNOSIS OF ADHD IN CHILDHOOD

■

The characteristics I have listed in Chapter 4 are those that describe ADHD children. The formal diagnosis is based on criteria published by the American Psychiatric Association in *Diagnostic and Statistical Manual of Mental Disorders*, 4th edition (DSM-IV).* This manual does not describe all the symptoms I have discussed, *only* those necessary to make the diagnosis of ADHD. The diagnostic criteria employed by clinicians in making the diagnosis are as follows.

A. The patient must have either symptoms of (1) inattention or (2) hyperactivity-impulsivity.
   1. *Inattention*: Six or more of the following symptoms of inattention have persisted for at least six months to a degree that is maladaptive and inconsistent with developmental level.
      a. Often fails to give close attention to details or makes careless mistakes in schoolwork, work, or other activities.

*Material reprinted with permission from the *Diagnostic and Statistical Manual of Mental Disorders*, 4th edition. Copyright 1994 American Psychiatric Association.

     b. Often has difficulty sustaining attention to tasks or play activities.

     c. Often does not seem to listen when spoken to directly.

     d. Often fails to follow through on instructions or complete schoolwork, chores, or duties (not due to a failure to understand instructions or being oppositional or negativistic).

     e. Often has difficulty organizing tasks and activities.

     f. Often avoids, dislikes, or is reluctant to engage in tasks that require sustained mental effort (such as schoolwork or homework).

     g. Often loses things necessary for tasks or activities (e.g., toys, school assignments, pencils, books).

     h. Is often easily distracted by outside stimuli.

     i. Is often forgetful in daily activities.

2. *Hyperactivity-impulsivity*: Six or more of the following symptoms of hyperactivity-impulsivity that have persisted for at least six months to a degree that is inconsistent with developmental level.

Hyperactivity

     a. Often fidgets with hands or feet or squirms in seat.

     b. Often leaves seat in classroom or in situations in which remaining seated is expected.

     c. Often runs about or climbs excessively in situations in which it is inappropriate (in adolescents or adults this may be limited to *feelings* of restlessness).

     d. Often has difficulty playing or engaging in leisure activities quietly.

     e. Is often "on the go" or often acts as if "driven by a motor."

     f. Often talks excessively.

Impulsivity

     g. Often blurts out answers to questions before they have been completed.

    h. Often has difficulty waiting turn.

    i. Often interrupts or intrudes on others (e.g., butts into conversations or games).

B. Some hyperactive-impulsive or inattention symptoms that caused impairment were present before age seven years.

C. Some impairment from the symptoms is present in two or more settings (e.g., at school or work and at home).

D. There must be clear evidence of clinically significant impairment in social, academic, or occupational functioning.

E. The symptoms of ADHD must not occur exclusively during the course of other psychiatric disorders such as psychotic disorders and are not better accounted for by other mental disorders such as mood disorder, anxiety disorder, or disorders of personality.

The characteristics listed are not meant to imply that these are the only symptoms that ADHD children have; they are the *minimal* symptoms necessary to make a diagnosis of the disorder. Needless to say, the rules cannot be followed mechanically but must be used by a clinician who has had training and experience in diagnosing childhood psychiatric disorders.

ADHD is divided into three categories:

1. *Attention-Deficit Hyperactivity Disorder, Combined Type*: If six or more symptoms of *inattentiveness* and six or more symptoms of *hyperactivity-impulsivity* have been present for the past six months, this diagnostic category is assigned.

2. *Attention-Deficit Hyperactivity Disorder, Predominantly Inattentive Type*: If six or more symptoms of inattention are met but fewer than six symptoms of hyperactivity-impulsivity are met, and these symptoms have been present for the past six months, this diagnosis is used.

3. *Attention-Deficit Hyperactivity Disorder, Predominantly Hyperactive Impulsive Type*: If six or more

symptoms of hyperactivity-impulsivity are present but fewer than six symptoms of inattention have been present for the past six months, this category is assigned.

These are the criteria by which a diagnosis of ADHD is made. DSM-IV also notes features that frequently accompany ADHD (many of which have been discussed earlier). These features vary with age and stage of development but include "low frustration tolerance, temper outbursts, bossiness, stubbornness, excessive and frequent insistence that requests be met, mood lability [instability]," "demoralization [feelings of ineffectuality and helplessness]," "dysphoria [feelings of dissatisfaction or discomfort]," and "rejection by peers and poor self-esteem."

It is also important to remember that ADHD may be accompanied by other psychiatric conditions, may resemble other psychiatric conditions (and thus be misdiagnosed as present when the other disorder is actually present), or hide behind other psychiatric disorders. This list includes, but is not limited to: Anxiety Disorder, Conduct Disorder, Depression, Learning Disorders, Obsessive Compulsive Disorder, Oppositional Defiant Disorder, Substance Abuse. The major features of Oppositional Defiant Disorder and Conduct Disorder are listed below.

OPPOSITIONAL DEFIANT DISORDER

A. A pattern of negativistic, hostile, and defiant behavior lasting at least six months, during which four (or more) of the following are present:
1. Often loses temper.
2. Often argues with adults.
3. Often actively defies or refuses to comply with adults' requests or rules.

4. Often deliberately annoys people.
5. Often blames others for his or her mistakes or misbehavior.
6. Is often touchy or easily annoyed by others.
7. Is often angry and resentful.
8. Is often spiteful or vindictive.
B. The disturbance in behavior causes clinically significant impairment in social, academic, or occupational functioning.
C. The behaviors do not occur exclusively during the course of a Psychotic or Mood Disorder.
D. Criteria are not met for Conduct Disorder (for children less than eighteen).

CONDUCT DISORDER

A. A more repetitive, and persistent pattern of behavior in which the basic rights of others or major age-appropriate rules are violated, as shown by the presence of three (or more) of the following criteria in the past twelve months, with at least one criterion present in the past six months:
   1. Aggression to people and animals.
   2. Destruction of property.
   3. Deceitfulness or theft.
   4. Serious violations of rules.
B. The disturbance in behavior causes clinically significant impairment in social, academic, or occupational functioning.

DIAGNOSIS OF ADHD
IN ADULTHOOD

■

The methods our research group employs to diagnose ADHD in adults are the "Utah Diagnostic Criteria," so called because they were devised by me and my colleagues at the University of Utah. They form the basis of the research we have done on adult ADHD during the past twenty-five years. When we began this research, it was the widely held belief that ADHD diminished in adolescence and disappeared in adulthood. Therefore, we decided to study the most clear-cut cases, adults who as children would have been diagnosed with ADHD, Combined Type. We have thus studied adults with more severe symptoms and a greater number of symptoms. Over time, we and others have found that some children with the purely inattentive form of ADHD grow up to be ADHD adults whose main symptom is inattention and that these adults often respond to treatment with medication, as do those adults with a number of symptoms. This form is not uncommon, but inattention is a common symptom of many psychiatric disorders. Now that we recognize the "full-fledged" form of ADHD in adults and have demonstrated its response to treatment, I anticipate that these milder forms of ADHD will be recognized as genuine variants of ADHD and will be the subject of further research on diagnosis and treatment. I must emphasize once again that the Utah Criteria evolved from our experience over many years and are provisional. We use them because they work. They will undoubtedly be modified by others and possibly replaced. For the present, we employ them as the most effective tool for the diagnosis of ADHD in adults.

THE UTAH CRITERIA FOR THE DIAGNOSIS OF
ADHD IN ADULTS

I. Childhood Characteristics
The first and most important point is that the individual must have had ADHD in childhood. We retrospectively diagnose ADHD in childhood in two ways:
   1. By contacting the mother or rearing person of the patient and directly inquiring about the symptoms that DSM-IV requires to make a definitive diagnosis of ADHD in childhood.
   2. By inquiring of the patient through administration of questionnaires for the retrospective diagnosis of ADHD in childhood.

The symptoms about which we inquire are as follows. The patient must have had both symptoms 1 and 2 and at least one other symptom from 3 to 6 in the following list:

1. *Attention problems.* Sometimes described as having a "short attention span," distractibility, unable to follow instructions in school or to complete schoolwork.
2. *Hyperactivity.* More active than other children, unable to sit still, fidgety, restless, always on the go, talking excessively.
3. *Impulsivity.*
4. *Behavior problems in school.*
5. *Overexcitability.*
6. *Temper outbursts.*

and

A high score on the rating scales, which measure the severity of ADHD symptoms in childhood. Those we have employed have been published in the author's book—directed at professionals—*Attention-Deficit Hyperactivity Disorder in Adults* (Oxford University Press, New York, 1995).

II. Adult Characteristics

In evaluating the adult, the presence of a spouse, partner, parent, or older sibling is of great value. As already mentioned, ADHD adults, having had the symptoms their entire life, are often blind to characteristics obvious to others.

The following are the seven major symptom groups we have found in the adults who clearly have ADHD in childhood and continued to have similar—and other—problems as adults. When we began our research in the early 1970s, the existence of "minimal brain dysfunction" (as ADHD was then called) in adults was not recognized and we elected to study those patients who had many clear-cut symptoms. After the publication of the first edition of the DSM, we followed its guidelines and studied patients, all of whom had problems with attention and continuing hyperactivity. (These patients would have qualified for a diagnosis of ADHD, Combined Type, if we had required symptoms of impulsivity as well.)

The diagnostic criteria that evolved were as follows. For an adult to have ADHD, he or she must have had symptoms 1 and 2 and two of symptoms 3 through 7 in the following list. If you do have this pattern, we would definitely diagnose you as having ADHD. And—in the tradition of medical jargon— we would diagnose you as having "classical" ADHD. In our experience, you should be evaluated.

As we and others have continued our studies, we have increasingly recognized adults who had childhood ADHD of the predominantly Inattentive Type and whose continuing problems are mainly in the areas of attention and disorganization. Although there are no scientific studies of this group of ADHD adults, it is our clinical experience that many of them respond favorably to the same drug treatments, as do the patients with "classical ADHD." A problem in diagnosing adult patients with ADHD, Inattentive Type, is that inattentiveness is a very nonspecific symptom.

Problems with attention occur in many other psychiatric disorders, and the evaluating psychiatrist will have to determine that the inattentiveness and disorganization are not symptoms of one of these disorders. Nonetheless, if you have symptoms of inattention and disorganization that are impairing your functioning, you should seek evaluation. We have not studied adults who had childhood ADHD of the Predominantly Hyperactive-Impulsive Type. It is quite likely that if you have symptoms of hyperactivity or impulsivity and two of the symptoms 3 through 6 that you have this variant of ADHD and should seek evaluation.

1. Attentional Difficulties

Characterized by an inability to keep one's mind on conversations (a frequent complaint of partners is that "he never listens to me and I have to repeat myself again and again"); distractibility (being aware of other stimuli when attempts are made to filter them out); difficulty keeping one's mind on reading materials or task; one's frequent "forgetfulness"; often losing or misplacing things (forgetting plans, car keys, purse, wallet, etc.); "mind frequently somewhere else."

2. Persistent Hyperactivity

Characterized by restlessness, inability to relax, "nervousness" (meaning an inability to settle down—not meaning anxious); inability to persist in sedentary activities (e.g., watching movies or TV, reading the newspaper); always being on the go, unhappy when inactive; talking excessively; fidgeting, often kicking or tapping foot.

3. Mood Instability

Usually described as beginning before adolescence and in some instances going as far back as the patient can remember. Definite shifts from a normal mood to depression or mild euphoria or—more often—excitement; depression described as being "down," "bored," or "discontented"; mood shifts usually last hours to at most a few days and are present without the physical symptoms of clinical depression; mood shifts may occur spontaneously but are usually in reaction to life experience. They can be prolonged if the patient must deal with-often self-engendered-difficult life experience.

4. Disorganization, Inability to Complete Tasks

The patient reports lack of organization on the job, running the household, or performing schoolwork; tasks frequently not completed; switches from one subject to another in a haphazard fashion; disorganization in activities, problem solving, keeping appointments, organizing time; lack of stick-to-it-iveness.

5. Hot Temper, Explosive Short-lived Outbursts

Patients reports outbursts may be accompanied by loss of control. Anger is not, however, persistent. Easily provoked or constant irritability. Easily irritated while driving (others don't start soon enough after the light turns green, are driving too slow, cutting in, etc.) Temper problems can obviously interfere with personal relationships.

6. Emotional Overreactivity

Patient cannot take ordinary stresses in stride and reacts excessively or inappropriately with depression, confusion, uncertainty, anxiety, or anger. Emotional responses interfere with appropriate problem solving. Subject experiences repeated crises in dealing with routine life events. May describe self as easily "hassled" or "stressed out."

7. Impulsivity

Minor symptoms include talking before thinking, interrupting other's conversations or finishing sentences for them, impatience (which contributes to driving problems), impulse buying, buying sprees. Subject makes decisions quickly and easily without reflection, often on the basis of insufficient information, to his or her own disadvantage; is unable to delay acting without discomfort. Major symptoms include hasty business or financial decisions, abrupt initiation or termination of relationships.

Features often associated with ADHD: marital instability; academic and vocational success less than expected given intelligence and education; substance abuse; histories of ADHD in children and other relatives.

ADHD AND OTHER PSYCHIATRIC DISORDERS

We have already mentioned the association of ADHD and Learning Disorders in childhood. It is probable that ADHD adults have an increased risk of having Learning Disorders as well. These are rarely inquired about or tested for but should certainly be investigated in underachieving students (including those without ADHD) and those ADHD subjects in whom problems in reading may underlie poor job performance. It is important to emphasize that other psychiatric problems may occur with adult ADHD, may mask it, or be misdiagnosed as ADHD. A very brief list of the more common conditions is given below. The correct diagnosis of ADHD requires investigation into all of these (and other) possible conditions.

Anxiety Disorders

Symptoms include chronic states of anxiety, worry, physiological arousal (sweaty palms, rapid heartbeat, tension headaches, upset stomach, etc.).

Bipolar Mood Disorders (formerly called manic-depressive disorder)

These illnesses may sometimes occur in relatively mild forms, where the ups and downs may somewhat resemble the mood instability seen in ADHD. Typically, when they occur in more extreme forms, they are more easily recognized and are accompanied by multiple symptoms, including physical ones.

Unipolar (One-sided) Depression ("Clinical Depression")

Symptoms include sadness, feeling down, an extensive loss of interest in and pleasure from formerly enjoyable activities; a loss of motivation; anxiety; guilt; suicidal thoughts; decreases in energy, sleep, sex drive, and appetite.

Personality Disorders

These disorders involve enduring characteristics of personality that result in individual unhappiness and frequently in social maladjustment. They have been present throughout the subject's life and, like ADHD, and for the same reason, may not be noticed by the subject. Different personality disorders may be characterized by impulsivity, difficulty in interpersonal relationships, hot temper, and an increased tendency to abuse substances. (To mention just a few of the problems seen.)

The take-home message is that adult ADHD is a condition for the experienced clinician to diagnose and is a diagnosis that can be suggested—but not conclusively made—using the criteria and rating scales alone.

PRESENTATION OF RATING SCALES

■

We have found that most patients cannot remember the exact symptoms of the DSM-IV criteria. The criteria require that some of the symptoms should have present before the age of seven and include items such as "often has difficulty playing or engaging in leisure activities quietly"; often has difficulty sustaining attention in tasks or play activities." When we compared adults' reports with rating scales to determine the presence of ADHD in childhood, we found that, in many instances, the patients' self-diagnoses were inaccurate. That is, many of these self-diagnosed patients did not have ADHD as based on the rating scales. When we administered medication to a group of ADHD patients, those who were self-diagnosed but had low scores on the rating scales failed to respond to medication, while those who had high scores did respond. This showed the reason for using these scales when we could not obtain direct histories from the patients' parents. In instances when parents were not available, we diagnosed the patients by a second method.

We would then ask patients about less specific symptoms and administer questionnaires for the retrospective diagnosis of ADHD in childhood.

PARENT'S RATING SCALE AND WENDER UTAH RATING SCALE (WURS)

The two rating scales we have employed in our research are the Parent's Rating Scale and the Wender Utah Rating Scale (WURS). As mentioned, we have found that possible ADHD

patients with high scores on the Patient's Rating Scale responded to drug treatment, while those with low scores did
not. It has apparently not been used frequently by clinicians
and researchers, although we have found most patients and
their parents are quite willing to have it employed. The
WURS is apparently being used increasingly by researchers
studying adult ADHD and has been translated into seven languages. It also seems that more and more clinicians are em-
ploying it.

The Parent's Rating Scale, reproduced below, is to be filled
out by the adult who served as the child's rearing figure. The
rating is made by assigning numbers to each of the 10 questions: not at all = 0; just a little = 1; pretty much = 2; very
much = 3. Since there are ten questions, the maximum score
is 30. A score of 12 indicates a high likelihood of ADHD in
childhood, while a score of 16 or higher indicates virtual cer-
tainty of ADHD in childhood.

Parents' Rating Scale

Patient's name _____ # _____ Date _____ Physician _____

To be filled out by the *mother* of the subject (or father only if mother is unavailable).

Instructions: Listed below are items concerning children's behavior and the problems they sometimes have. Read each item carefully and decide how much you think your child was bothered by these problems when he/she was between *six* and *ten* years old. Enter the amount of the problem by putting a check in the column that describes your child at that time.

		NOT AT ALL	JUST A LITTLE	PRETTY MUCH	VERY MUCH
1.	RESTLESS (OVERACTIVE)				
2.	EXCITABLE, IMPULSIVE				
3.	DISTURBS OTHER CHILDREN				
4.	FAILS TO FINISH THINGS STARTED (SHORT ATTENTION SPAN)				
5.	FIDGETING				
6.	INATTENTIVE, DISTRACTIBLE				
7.	DEMANDS MUST BE MET IMMEDIATELY; GETS FRUSTRATED				
8.	CRIES				
9.	MOOD CHANGES QUICKLY				
10.	TEMPER OUTBURSTS (EXPLOSIVE AND UNPREDICTABLE BEHAVIOR)				

From Paul H. Wender, *Attention-Deficit Hyperactivity Disorder in Adults* (New York: Oxford University Press, 1995).

A score of 12 indicates that the patient would have been in the 95th percentile for ADHD in childhood; that is, among the upper 5 percent.

WENDER UTAH RATING SCALE (WURS)

PATIENT'S INITIALS _____ PATIENT'S NUMBER _____ DATE _____ M.D.'s INITIALS _____

AS A CHILD I WAS (OR HAD):	Not at all or very slightly	Mildly	Moder-ately	Quite a Bit	Very Much
1. Active, restless, always on the go					
2. Afraid of things					
3. Concentration problems, easily distracted					
4. Anxious, worrying					
5. Nervous, fidgety					
6. Inattentive, daydreaming					
7. Hot or short tempered, low boiling point					
8. Shy, sensitive					
9. Temper outbursts, tantrums					
10. Trouble with stick-to-it-tiveness, not following through, failing to finish things started					
11. Stubborn, strong willed					
12. Sad or blue, depressed, unhappy					
13. Uncautious, dare-devilish, involved in pranks					
14. Not getting a kick out of things, dissatisfied with life					
15. Disobedient with parents, rebellious, sassy					
16. Low opinion of myself					
17. Irritable					
18. Outgoing, friendly, enjoy company of people					
19. Sloppy, disorganized					
20. Moody, have ups and downs					
21. Feel angry					
22. Have friends, popular					
23. Well organized, tidy, neat					
24. Acting without thinking, impulsive					
25. Tend to be immature					
26. Feel guilty, regretful					
27. Lose control of myself					
28. Tend to be or act irrational					
29. Unpopular with other children, didn't keep friends for long, didn't get along with other children					
30. Poorly coordinated, did not participate in sports					

From Paul H. Wender, *Attention-Deficit Hyperactivity Disorder in Adults* (New York: Oxford University Press, 1995).

AS A CHILD I WAS (OR HAD):	Not at all or very slightly	Mildly	Moderately	Quite a Bit	Very Much
31. Afraid of losing control of self					
32. Well coordinated, picked first in games					
33. (for women only) Tomboyish					
34. Ran away from home					
35. Get in fights					
36. Teased other children					
37. Leader, bossy					
38. Difficulty getting awake					
39. Follower, lead around too much					
40. Trouble seeing things from someone else's point of view					
41. Trouble with authorities, trouble with school, visits to principal's office					
42. Trouble with the police, booked, convicted					
MEDICAL PROBLEMS AS A CHILD:					
43. Headaches					
44. Stomachaches					
45. Constipation					
46. Diarrhea					
47. Food allergies					
48. Other allergies					
49. Bedwetting					
AS A CHILD IN SCHOOL:					
50. Overall a good student, fast					
51. Overall a poor student, slow learner					
52. Slow reader					
53. Slow in *learning* to read					
54. Trouble reversing letters					
55. Problems with spelling					
56. Trouble with mathematics or numbers					
57. Bad handwriting					
58. Though I could read pretty well, I never really enjoyed reading					
59. Did not achieve up to potential					
60. Repeated grades (which grades?) _____					
61. Suspended or expelled (which grades?)					

Source: Paul H. Wender, M.D., University of Utah School of Medicine, Salt Lake City, UT 84132.

Scoring: Not at all   = 0.
       Mildly   = 1.
       Moderately = 2.
       Quite a bit = 3.
       Very much = 4.

In scoring the WURS, each response carries a number: not at all or very slightly = 0; mildly = 1; moderately = 2; quite a bit = 3; very much = 4. The score is determined by totaling the response numbers for all of the questions. The average score for ADHD adults is 62; the average score for normal subjects is 16.

Of normal adults, 95 percent obtain a score of 34 or lower and 99 percent obtain a score of 41 or lower. That means that with a score of 34 it is very likely that an adult had ADHD in childhood and with a score of 41 or more it is extremely probable. However, other childhood conditions may also receive high scores, so that the clinician must be certain that the patient who is being evaluated did not have one of these disorders. Similarly, some children who appeared to have ADHD in childhood develop other disorders as adults. This means that a full clinical evaluation must explore the possibility of whether or not another psychiatric disorder is present.

In conclusion, having read this book, if you feel you meet the symptom requirements for ADHD or have many of the symptoms listed, you may have adult ADHD. However, a correct and precise diagnosis must be made by an adult psychiatrist who can determine if you do indeed have adult ADHD or another psychiatric disorder.

Index

■